Epidemiology of Cancer of Selected Sites in Poland and Polish Migrants

The preparation and publication of this monograph was supported through the Special Foreign Currency Program of the National Library of Medicine, National Institutes of Health, Public Health Service, U.S. Department of Health, Education and Welfare, Bethesda, Maryland, under an agreement with the Coordinating Commission for Polish-American Scientific Collaboration to the Scientific Council to the Minister of Health and Social Welfare, Government of Poland, Warsaw.

Epidemiology of Cancer of Selected Sites in Poland and Polish Migrants

Jerzy Staszewski

Ballinger Publishing Company. Cambridge, Mass.
A Subsidiary of J. B. Lippincott Company

Library of Congress Catalog Card Number 74-1096
International Standard Book Number 0-88410-114-2

Library of Congress Cataloging in Publication Data
STASZEWSKI JERZY.
   Epidemiology of cancer of selected sites in Poland and Polish migrants.

   1. Cancer—Poland—Statistics. 2. Epidemiology.
I. Title. (DNML; 1. Neoplasma—Etiology.
2. Neoplasma—Occurrence—Poland. QZ200 S796e 1974/
RC279.P7S7   614.5′999′09438   74-1096
ISBN 0-88410-114-2

Printed in Poland

Foreword

Much of data reported in Dr. Staszewski's monograph was collected in studies undertaken jointly by the Oncological Institutes (Poland) and the National Cancer Institute (United States). Financial support was received from the Special Foreign Currency (Public Law 480) Program, the medical research component of which is directed by the Coordinating Commission for the Polish-American Scientific Collaboration and the National Institutes of Health. Funds through the Public Law 480 Program for the preparation and publication of the present monograph were awarded as a part of the National Library of Medicine's Health Research Communication Program in Poland.

One motivation for work was the assembly of baseline data on cancer risks for comparison with the experience of Polish migrants to the United States and other countries. The migration of human populations is an experiment of nature that provides us with a tool that enables us to study the role of host and environmental factors in the development of disease. Cancer was the first group of diseases to be investigated systematically from this point of view and the current data from Poland will contribute to the existing pool of information on this subject. In years past the profile of site-specific cancer risks in Poland differed markedly from that prevailing in western Europe and the United States; for example, incidence and mortality from cancer of the breast and the large bowel have been far lower than in other countries. The risks for these sites among the Polish-born in the United States now approach those of the host population, which strongly suggests the intervention of environmental factors.

Effects similar to those observed for Polish migrants are now being detected within Poland and Dr. Staszewski describes a transition in risks for breast, colon and other sites to levels more closely approximating those in western Europe and North America. The appearance of a transitional phase means that ongoing work in Poland should be pursued, since observations on populations in transition are more likely to detect and pinpoint the factors responsible than studies carried out in populations with a more or less constant and homogeneous background of risks.

Since cancer is a group of diseases found in all races and ages of man, it is appropriate that cancer be international in scope and involve close cooperation among scientists from many countries. The present volume stimulated by a collaborative international effort suggests promising leads that would not have been easily uncovered by investigators working alone in their own countries.

WILLIAM HAENSZEL
Biometry Branch
National Cancer Institute
Bethesda, Maryland, U.S.A

Acknowledgements

To Mr. William Haenszel, Chief of the Biometry Branch of the National Cancer Institute, National Institutes of Health, Bethesda, Md., I am greatly indebted for inspiring my interest in the problem of cancer in migrant populations, for his help in obtaining unpublished data on Polish-born Americans, and for his most helpful comments and suggestions in the preparation of this monograph. I owe my sincerest gratitude to him and to Professor Dr. Hanna Kołodziejska, Director, Institute of Oncology of the Kraków Branch, to Professor Dr. Tadeusz Koszarowski, Director of the Institute of Oncology in Warszawa, to Professor Dr. Witold Niepołomski, Head of the Anatomo-Pathological Department of the Silesian Medical School in Katowice, and to Docent Dr. Jeremi Święcki, Director, Institute of Oncology of the Gliwice Branch, for their most kind encouragement and assistance, which enabled me to complete this monograph.

The Department of Vital Statistics and Demographic Studies of the Central Statistical Office in Warszawa provided unpublished tabulations of cancer mortality in Poland.

Directors of the Department, Mr. Zygmunt Zaremba, M. A. and Mr. Marian Klimczyk, M. A., as well as Mrs. Henryka Bogacka, M. A., were always most kind and helpful, for which I wish to express my appreciation.

The National Center for Health Statistics, Washington, D.C., supplied unpublished data on cancer mortality among Polish-born and native white Americans. Doctors Michael McCall and Norman Stenhouse, from Western Australia University, Perth, provided unpublished data on mortality among Polish migrants in Australia.

Some of the technical work, including computation and preparation of the drawings, was performed under PL-480 Agreement 05-009-01, sponsored by the National Cancer Institute, National Institutes of Health, Bethesda, Md.

The International Agency for Research on Cancer, Lyon, provided a desk calculator and helped in completing references. The chapters on alimentary tract cancer were reviewed by Dr. Calum S. Muir, Chief of the Unit of Epidemiology and Biostatistics of the Agency. I wish to express my gratitude for his kind interest and advice.

A part of this work was carried out under a fellowship from the Silesian Medical School in Katowice.

The publication of this monograph has been made possible with the support of the National Library of Medicine, Bethesda, Md.

Contents

List of Tables

Text Tables

Appendix Tables

List of Figures

Text Figures

Appendix Figures

1 | Introduction

1.1. Aims of the Present Study

The purpose of this monograph is to present and analyze the occurrence of cancer of the most important primary localization in Poland, looking out for implications for cancer etiopathogenesis. Based primarily on mortality statistics, the results will be put in proper perspective through comparison with mortality in other populations, including Polish migrants, as well as with cancer morbidity data.

1.2. Purpose, Directions and Significance of Cancer Epidemiology and Etiopathogenesis Studies

Cancer epidemiology is concerned not only with ascertaining cancer occurrence, but also with detecting those factors which determine this occurrence and bear on cancer risk: in other words — with cognition of cancer etiopathogenesis.

Factors favoring cancer genesis, increasing cancer risk, will be called **carcinogenic factors.** This is a broad term, covering not only the initiating and promoting factors (carcinogens and co-carcinogens), but also habits, customs, demographic and occupational characteristics such as tobacco smoking, working in uranium mines, and the like, which are connected with an increased cancer risk.

Both epidemiologic observations and animal experiments demonstrate that the same type of cancer can be produced by a large variety of carcinogenic factors or their complexes. For example, skin cancer can be produced by the carcinogenic hydrocarbons, by arsenic, or by the sun rays (more common in persons with fair complexion). Some such factors may predominate, as in the case of cigarette smoking in lung cancer genesis.

Under suitable conditions, cancer can be produced either by a single action or by the long-term influence of a carcinogenic factor, an example of the former situation being the irradiation at an atomic bomb explosion, and of the latter, tobacco smoking. The time interval between the beginning of the action of carcinogenic factors and the appearance of cancer symptoms is long, usually two or more decades. This renders the identification of even a single carcinogenic factor much more difficult. Such identification is even more difficult when a complex of carcinogenic factors operates, partly because the individual factors of such a complex may be acting at different times, and partly because cancer may develop even in the absence of some of the factors of this complex.

These observations, together with the applied definition of carcinogenic factors, point to the conclusion that the frequency of cancer occurrence in a population depends on the prevalence, intensity and co-operation of carcinogenic factors. Cancers of different tissues and organs do not necessarily depend on the same carcinogenic factors. For example, exposure to aniline dyes increases the risk of urinary bladder cancer, whereas exposure to asbestos — the risk of mesothelioma and lung cancer. Localisation of the carcinogenic effect of a chemical carcinogen may be determined by its portal of entry, site of localisation, metabolism or excretion.

Carcinogenic factors may be divided into **environmental** (exogenous) and **host** (endogenous) factors. It should be kept in mind, however, that the host factors are not necessarily genetic, but may also depend on environmental factors such as nutrition, previous history of diseases and the like. As **genetic factors** will be considered both the disposition characteristic of a genus, species or race which leads to regional or racial differences in cancer occurrence (such as differences in skin cancer occurrence related to racial variation in skin pigmentation), as well as familial disposition, exemplified by the familial intestinal polyposis.

Differentiation between the effects of genetic and environmental factors is difficult. For example, the more frequent occurrence of some type of cancer in certain families might be ascribed to either the familial genetic disposition or to familial similarities in habits, customs and environment. Ethnic differences in cancer occurrence likewise may depend on either genetic factors or environment, habit and custom characteristics. One of the principal objectives of epidemiologic studies is the evaluation of the relative importance of environmental and genetic factors as determinants of the frequency of cancer occurrence.

Two main avenues of epidemiological research may be distinguished: descriptive and analytical.

Descriptive epidemiology, also called geographic pathology, is concerned with cancer occurrence in individual populations and time periods, as well as with trends and regional differences in cancer occurrence. Studies of this type so far published in Poland have been based on autopsy statistics — e.g.: Ciechanowski; Kulig et al. [28,105], on mortality statistics — e.g.: Bielecki and Piekutowska; Krasuska; Staszewski [17,102,169,170], and on incidence data from registration statistics — e.g.: Kołodziejska; Koszarowski et al. [88,91,97,98,100].

The purpose of **analytical epidemiology** is to explain epidemiological phenomena established by the epidemiologic description, as well as to search for factors bearing on cancer risk. The starting point is, as a rule, the results of descriptive epidemiology.

The two most important methods of cancer analytical epidemiology are the case-control and cohort studies.

Case-control or **retrospective studies** consist of gathering information about exposure to the factors under study both from persons with the investigated disease (study group) and from individuals without that disease who constitute a control or comparison group. Comparison of both groups permits evaluation of the relationship between the study factors and the investigated disease.

Case-control studies may be concerned with a specific factor such as smoking or be designed to find factors bearing on cancer risk. Such studies were and are conducted in Poland on cancer of the gastro-intestinal tract, cancer of the breast and uterus, and on the relationship between smoking and cancer [164,167,174,178,179]; their results will be cited in the following chapters.

Cohort or **prospective studies** consist of collecting similar information from persons without the cancer under study and of their subsequent follow-up for many years. Occurrence of the investigated disease can then be established in relation to various levels of exposure to the factors under study. Prospective studies are very expensive, and thus have to be directed to testing specific hypotheses; no such studies have been conducted in Poland. The methodology, underlying assumptions, and aims of case-control and cohort studies are discussed in detail by Lilienfeld, Pedersen and Dowd [109]; MacMahon, Pugh and Ipsen [116]; and Mantel and Haenszel [117].

Results of epidemiologic studies may have both cognitive and practical value. Knowledge of the frequency, demographic characteristics and time trends of cancer occurrence is important to the organization and planning of the campaign against cancer and to the formulation and checking of hypotheses about cancer etiopathogenesis. Detection of carcinogenic factors and determination of their mode of action not only enriches our knowledge, but also may lead to effective cancer prophylaxis through the elimination of the detected carcinogenic factor. Knowledge of changes in cancer occurrence after such prophylactic action may help in the evaluation of its effectiveness.

Initially, epidemiologic studies concerning cancer were sporadic and usually limited to occupational cancers. For example, in 1775 Pott described the frequent occurrence of scrotal cancer among chimney sweepers [133], which preceded for many decades both the experimental demonstration of the carcinogenity of soot and the isolation of benzpyrene and other carcinogenic hydrocarbons. A more rapid development of cancer epidemiology studies took place in recent decades, especially after the Second World War.

A few examples of the results of cancer epidemiology studies using mortality statistics will be shown in the following subchapter. A more detailed discussion of the methods, results and applications of epidemiologic studies are presented by Kostrzewski and Brzeziński [92]; Lilienfeld, Pedersen and Dowd [109], and MacMahon, Pugh and Ipsen [116].

1.3. Mortality Statistics in the Study of Cancer Epidemiology

The high value of mortality statistics for epidemiologic research is demonstrated not only by theoretical considerations, but also by past experience. It is even stated that "... the statistics of a large number of countries permit studies of the relationship between the various forms of cancer and age, sex, marital status, and social class, in addition to the variables, previously discussed. It is safe to state that nearly all that is known regarding their relation to cancer has originally been established, or at least suggested, by studies of routinely available official mortality data" [109].

Analyses of cancer mortality statistics have made possible the detection of many epidemiologic phenomena, such as differences in the risk of cancers in specific parts of the body between different populations or changes in those risks over time. Such analyses have also helped to formulate and test epidemiologic hypotheses. As early as 1842, Rigioni Stern analysed mortality in Verona in the 1760–1839 period and demonstrated a higher frequency of breast cancer among unmarried females, specifically nuns, than among married — the opposite of the behavior of uterine cancer [189].

Analyses of mortality statistics in England and Wales [118,197] demonstrated the relationship of cancer occurrence to occupation and socioeconomic class. For example, a high mortality from cancer of the buccal cavity, pharynx and esophagus was demonstrated among persons who are occupationally exposed to alcoholic beverages; the association between alcohol consumption and the risk of these cancers was corroborated by case-control studies [210].

Studies of lung cancer mortality demonstrated a large increase in mortality rates, much more rapid for males than for females. Pecularities in geographic distribution were also noted, including a high mortality in Great Britain and Finland, and a low one in Norway and Iceland. These observations have not only awakened interest in lung cancer and led to the well known studies of its relation to tobacco smoking and air pollution, but also helped in checking hypotheses on the etiopathogenesis of this cancer [165].

Variations in leukemia and thyroid cancer mortality led to investigation of the harmfulness of the "prophylactic" infant thymus irradiation, a praxis popular in the United States. Cessation of such irradiation was followed by a decrease of leukemia mortality among children [26,50].

Another example of the utilization of mortality statistics for epidemiologic research is the comparative studies made of cancer risk among first and second generation migrants to the United States [60,65] which, for example, helped to evaluate the relative importance of environmental and genetic factors in cancer etiopathogenesis. Mortality statistics were utilized to determine the dependence of lung cancer risk not only upon the place of last residence, but also upon the place of birth [67]; the provocative results, suggesting new avenues in research of lung cancer etiopathogenesis, will be discussed in Chapter 8.

1.4. Some General Data about Poland*

Poland is located in Central Europe, between the 49°00′ and 54°50′ parallels North and between 14°07′ and 24°08′ longitude East. It borders the U.S.S.R. on the East, Czechoslovakia on the South and the German Democratic Republic on the West. Most of the northern Polish border is formed by the Baltic Sea — the drainage basin of 99.8 percent of the area of Poland. The borders of Poland roughly resemble a circle (Figure 1-1).

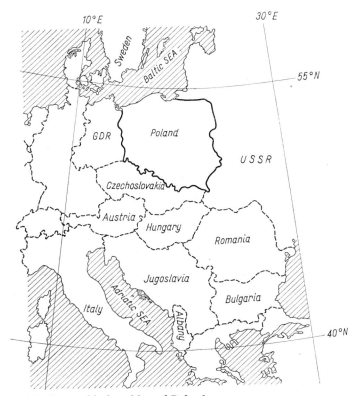

Fig. 1-1. Geographical position of Poland.

Poland is definitely a low-lying country. Seventy five percent of its area is no higher than 200 meters above sea level, and only 2.7 percent is higher than 500 meters above sea level. Average altitude is 174 meters above sea level.

Poland is located in the temperate climate zone, influenced mainly by oceanic air masses coming from Western and Northern Europe (about 60 percent of the prevailing winds come from the west) but also by continental air masses from Eastern Europe. Average annual precipitation is about 600 milimeters. Average

* Based on *Polish Statistical Yearbooks*, on publications of the results of population censuses [18,129,138,139,140], and on the article "Polska" (Poland) in the *Great General Encyclopedia (Wielka Encyklopedia Powszechna)*, vol. 9, PWN, Warszawa, 1967.

annual temperature (including readings from various regions of the country, with the exception of the mountains) ranges from 6° to 9° centigrade. The average temperatures of the coldest month (January) and the warmest (July), respectively, range from 0° to — 4.5° centigrade, and from 16.5° to 19° centigrade.

The area of Poland is close to 313,000 square kilometers; its population as of December 31, 1970, is 32,600,000; and the average density of population is 104 persons per square kilometer.

Administratively, Poland was divided * into 17 districts ("voivodship"), in Polish "województwo", and 5 metropolitan cities (Warszawa, Kraków, Łódź, Poznań, Wrocław) which had the same status as the districts (Figure 1-2). The districts were divided into counties, in Polish "powiat", of which there were 463.

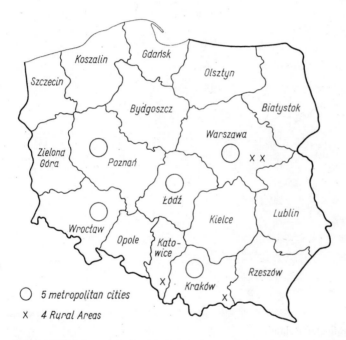

Fig. 1-2. Division of Poland into administrative Districts and location of the regional cancer registries.

Several regions of Poland display some characteristic demographic features. For example, the most industrial is the Katowice District, discussed in more detail on page 11. On the other extreme, the Eastern Districts (Rzeszów, Lublin, Białystok) are characterized by the highest percentage of the rural population (over 60 percent) and of the agricultural population (over 43 percent). The Western Territories (Districts of Wrocław, Zielona Góra, Szczecin and Koszalin) have the highest percentage of the immigratory population; population shifts during and

* up to 1974.

after the last World War, directed mostly from East to West, affected the present population of these territories more than the population of the other areas of Poland. Moreover, the average age of the population of the Western Territories is lower than that of the population of the other regions. Compared with other regions, the percentage of individuals under the age of 19 is highest in the Western Territories, and the percentage of those 65 and over, is lowest.

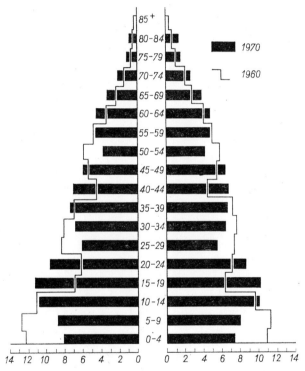

Fig. 1-3. Structure of the population of Poland, by sex and age, according to the 1960 and 1970 censuses.

The population of Poland is homogeneous with respect to nationality. In 1960, the non-Polish population was estimated at about 450,000 (1.5 percent of the total population), of which about 350,000 were Ukrainians and White Russians. The population of Poland is also relatively young. The percentage of individuals below the age of 19 is one of the highest in Europe (40.2 percent in 1960, 37.0 percent in 1970); and of older people, aged 65 and over, is one of the lowest (6.9 percent in 1960, and 8.5 percent in 1970). The population structure by age and sex, as established by the general population censuses of 1960 and 1970, is presented in Figure 1-3 and in Appendix Table A-1.

As a result of post-war industrialization, Poland has been transformed from an agricultural country into an industrial one. That part of the population making its living from agriculture decreased from 60 percent in 1931 to 47 percent in 1950, to 38 percent in 1960, to 30 percent in 1970. The percentage of the population living in rural areas decreased from 73 in 1931 to 63 in 1950, to 52 in 1960, to 48 in 1970. Among industrial employees in 1965, 29 percent were engaged in the metal and machine industries, 12 percent in the food industry, 11 percent in the fuel industry, and 11 percent in the textile industry.

2 | Materials

2.1. Polish Cancer Mortality and Population Data

The detailed *International Classification of Diseases — ICD*, seventh, 1955 revision [120] — was first introduced in Poland in 1959, but since 1970 the eighth, 1965 revision of ICD has been used in Polish mortality statistics. Earlier mortality statistics, for the years 1951–1958, used only 10 classes for cancer and are not comparable with post–1958 data. Since the most recent data available for the preparation of this monograph were those for 1969, only the 1959–1969 period will be analyzed. Data for 1970 and 1971, obtained recently, were considered in analyzing time trends (Figures 4-15 and 4-16).

All the cancer mortality rates, some of which are shown in Appendix Tables 7-12 and 18, are computed from unpublished tabulations of cancer deaths by primary site, sex, age and residence provided by the Department of Vital Statistics and Demographic Studies, Central Statistical Office. Population estimates, used for computation of rates, were also provided by that Department.

Characteristics of Polish mortality statistics and of population estimates by age and residence have been presented in Polish [78,199,200], and are briefly summarized below.

Death certification in Poland follows the rules internationally accepted and recommended by the World Health Organization [120]. The death certificate, containing a statement on the cause of death, is usually issued by a physician (see Chapter 4.8 where the reliability of these statements is also discussed). Death certificates are collected, coded and processed by the Central Statistical Office.

Registration of deaths in Poland is believed to be complete. "The laws in force in Poland forbid burial without registration of the death certificate at the local registrar's office. Rigorous interpretation of these laws has resulted in death registration in Poland being complete and information on the demographic characteristics of the deceased reliable" [78]. Of those demographic characteristics, sex, age and residence will be considered in the present study. With respect to the last characteristic, Polish mortality statistics follow the accepted practice of classifying the deceased by the place of last residence rather than by place of death.

Classification of the population by residence will be made in two ways: one is based on the regional division of the country into administrative Districts (17 Districts and 5 metropolitan cities — see Chapter 1.4); the other is by the urban-rural character of the place of residence. Here the administrative criteria are followed: "... division of the population into urban or rural results from the legal character of their place of residence" [78].

2.2. Polish Cancer Incidence Data

Nationwide reporting of cancer has been compulsory in Poland since 1952. However, it has been found that given the resources available it has not been possible to obtain data of uniformly good quality from a central registration scheme covering the whole of the country, with a population of over 30 million.

Although the regulation to report cancer has not been revoked, nor has central registration ceased, special efforts have been made to improve the quality of registration in a few selected areas, where regional registries have been established with the support of the National Cancer Institute of the National Institutes of Health of the United States. These regional registries cover about 25 percent of the total urban and 16 percent of the total rural population of Poland. The report cards used are the same for all the regions, as are the codes used to process the data [94]. The location of these registries can be seen on Figure 1-2.

Information on cancer morbidity in Poland, presented in Appendix Tables 3, 4, 5, 6 and discussed in subsequent chapters, is derived from cancer registration in 1965–66 in the four selected regions: Warszawa City, Katowice District, Kraków Region (consisting of Kraków City and Kraków District), and 4 Rural Areas (consisting of the towns and counties of Cieszyn, Nowy Sącz, Mińsk Mazowiecki and Siedlce).

It is not known to what extent these regions are representative of the total population of Poland with respect to cancer occurrence, and all comparisons with mortality data pertaining to the whole country should be made with caution.

From the same UICC publication [41] in which these Polish cancer incidence data are published, data on cancer incidence in other countries, utilized for comparisons with Poland, are also derived. They too pertain, as a rule, to selected regions or population groups only, except for the Scandinavian countries, Scotland, Israel, and Puerto Rico.

Some data on the regions, where the Polish cancer registries mentioned above are operating, are presented below.

Warszawa City [95], the capital of Poland, is situated in the Mazovian Lowland. The area under registration totals 427 square kilometres. In 1965, the population was 1,252,600. The main occupational groups were: industry, 29.5 percent; education and culture, 12.4 percent; building construction, 11.2 percent; trade, 10.8 percent. With regard to medical services, there were 5,898 physicians and 32 hospitals with 12,435 beds, including 333 for cancer patients.

Katowice District [177,206] is the smallest of all the districts in Poland (3.1 percent of the total area) but has the largest population (3.5 million or 11 percent of the total). It is also the most urbanized and industrialized district, 76 percent of the population being urban. Fifty percent of the population derives its income from industry, only 9 percent from agriculture — whereas for the total country these proportions are respectively 50 percent and 34 percent. More than one-third of all industrial workers are engaged in coal mining. Steel and zinc smelting and other metallurgy, coking plants, chemical industry, electricity plants and machine manufacture are the other main industries.

The most heavily industrialized part of Katowice District is the GOP ("Górno-śląski Okręg Przemysłowy"), the Upper Silesia Industrial Area — a complex of several cities (conurbation), with very heavy air pollution, where 1,758,000 people or half of the population of this district live on 785 square kilometres.

The transportation network is well developed, a fact which contributes to easy access to medical care and to oncological centres, which are also quantitatively above the average for the whole country, there being 100 hospitals, 29,000 hospital beds and 4649 physicians (1967). Cieszyn City and County, which comprise 3.5 percent of the population of the Katowice District, were excluded from the data on cancer incidence for this District and included among the rural areas discussed below.

Kraków Region [89], consisting of the City of Kraków and the Kraków District (excluding Nowy Sącz city and county), is situated in the South of Poland. Of its approximately 2.5 million population (about 20 percent of which live in the city of Kraków), 56 percent are considered to be rural, but the majority work in industry or in the building trades and only about one-third earn a living from agriculture. In 1965, there were a total of 53 hospitals, including sanatoria, and over 16,000 beds as well as 3650 physicians in practice.

Four Rural Areas. The location of these areas is shown in Figure 1-2. Because the populations-at-risk are rather small, the data for these areas have been combined in the tables. These four areas are: Mińsk Mazowiecki County, Siedlce County and City, the Cieszyn area and the Nowy Sącz area. Their brief characteristics are presented below [90].

Mińsk and Siedlce Counties are located in the plains some 40 to 80 kilometers to the East of Warszawa. Seventy-one percent of the population is considered to be rural. The four cities in these counties, whose populations range from 1600 to 36,000, have a rural rather than an urban character. The principal occupation is farming. There is some light, but no heavy industry.

Medical care is provided by local health centres and hospitals. For diseases such as cancer, patients are referred to specialized centres in Warszawa for further investigation and treatment.

Cieszyn area, consisting of the city and county of Cieszyn, is located in the southern part of Katowice District. Whereas most of Katowice District is plain, part of Cieszyn County is highland. Only about 40 percent of the population lives in the five cities of the area, the largest having a population of 25,000, whereas 76 percent of the Katowice District population is urban.

The Cieszyn area is less industrialized than the rest of the Katowice District, and differs in the type of industry. Instead of heavy industry, wood and food production predominate, although there is also some manufacture of textiles, tools and electrical goods. Migration to and from this area is less than in the rest of the Katowice District. It is estimated that 90–95 percent of the inhabitants seek medical care within the area, permitting efficient and reliable checking of completeness in cancer reporting.

Nowy Sącz area, consisting of the city and county of Nowy Sącz, located in the southern part of the Kraków District, is geographically a distinct region consisting of a valley passing into highlands, largely separated by mountains from other regions. It has a highland climate.

About 66 percent of the population live in rural areas, the remainder in one of the six cities, of which Nowy Sącz with a population of 38,00 is the largest. Migration to and from the area is light. Farming is the main occupation — 61.5 percent of the population compared to 42.7 percent in the Kraków District. In constrast to the rest of the Kraków District, there is no heavy industry, only the production of wood and food.

The well-developed local health service and the geographical configuration prevent people from seeking medical care in the neighbouring counties. These factors help to maintain good cancer registration in the area.

2.3. Cancer Mortality Data from other Countries

Comparisons of cancer mortality between Poland and other countries will be based on cancer mortality rates in 1964–65 in 24 countries, published by Segi et al. [161]. Time trends in cancer mortality in the 1959–1969 period in Poland will be compared with time trends in the 1950—1965 period in the same 24 countries, presented by Segi et al. numerically and graphically for 1950–1963 [160], and numerically for 1964–65 [161]. These sources divide the United States population into "whites" and "nonwhites". Ninety percent of the latter are blacks; the balance are Asians and American Indians.

2.4. Cancer Mortality among Polish Migrants

Of necessity, comparisons of cancer mortality in Poland and among Polish migrants will be limited to the data on migrants to the United States of America and, to a smaller extent, Australia; despite some efforts, the author could obtain no access to detailed cancer mortality data on Polish migrants in any other country.

Unpublished sex- and age-specific cancer mortality rates for Polish-born Americans, made available by the National Center for Health Statistics of the Public Health Service, Washington, D.C., for 1950 — partly described in [180] — and for 1959–61, are presented in Appendix Tables 13, 14, 15, along with the rates for native white Americans. These last data, derived from the same source, will be used as a second set of reference values, besides those for Poland, for analyses of cancer mortality among Polish-born Americans.

The 1962–66 age-specific cancer mortality rates among Polish migrants to Australia are presented in Appendix Table 16. Comparison of these rates with data from the analogous period for both Poland and Australia is presented in another paper [181]. Mortality rates for Polish migrants to Australia provide further background data for the analyses of cancer mortality in Polish-born Americans; but they can be used for comparisons only for the most common types of cancer, because they are based on such small numbers — altogether only 460 cancer deaths among Polish migrants to Australia. For the same reason, age-specific rates for ages below 40 and over 80 will not be graphically presented for the migrants to Australia.

2.5. Comparison of the Advantages and Disadvantages of Cancer Mortality and Morbidity Statistics

The subsequent analyses of cancer occurrence will be based almost exclusively on mortality and morbidity statistics. Hence, a comparison of the advantages and disadvantages of both these sources of information as estimates of cancer risk is indicated.

1. On the death certificate more than one cause of death is often given, but in routine mortality statistics only one, sometimes arbitrally selected, is used — that one which is called the underlying cause. Special studies, however, such as one made in the United States, demonstrated that when cancer appears on death certificates in about 95 percent of cases it is as the underlying cause [42]. Therefore, in spite of the omission of a few cases of cancer reported as the contributory cause, not much is lost of the total information about cancer given on death certificates. Rules for qualification of causes of death, whether underlying or contributory, are laid down by the International Classification of Diseases [120], compulsory in Poland and in those other countries whose data will be used for comparison.

2. Information acquired from death certificates is less precise than data obtainable from cancer registries; for example information on the histologic type of cancer is not generally given on death certificates.

3 Epidemiology...

3. For cancers with a low fatality rate, like skin cancer, mortality data are of little value as measures of cancer risk, compared to incidence data.

4. Differences in treatment results may distort estimates of differentials in cancer risks based on mortality. However, the comparison of survival rates in six countries * showed that between-country variation in treatment policies had little bearing on cancer survival and could not explain the observed mortality differences [79].

5. Death is a well defined event occurring at a precise time — unlike the beginning of illness or date of the onset of symptoms.

6. Each death is usually reported — and reported only once. On the other hand, in morbidity statistics the same individual may be reported from several sources, a factor which creates problems in data processing. An individual with cancer, moreover, may not be reported at all, as is shown by the number of cases recorded for the first time on the basis of a death certificate in many cancer registries [41].

7. Comparability of data is best when their level of quality is similar. As a rule, this requirement is better met by mortality statistics. Doll states that "... in some areas in which cancer registration is incomplete, mortality can provide a better indication of incidence than the official "incidence statistics", particularly for cancers whose fatality is high..." [39].

8. The relatively steady level of the quality of mortality data permits better time-trend analyses.

9. Cancer mortality statistics are not very sensitive to such factors as mass surveys, which temporarily can markedly distort incidence data and patterns [181].

10. Good mortality statistics are available for the total populations of many countries with breakdowns by important demographic characteristics that facilitate meaningful international comparisons in spite of large differences in demographic structure. Comprehensive studies of cancer mortality statistics, taking into consideration such characteristics as sex, age, marital status, occupation, socioeconomic class, residence, regional differences and time trends, have been conducted in the United States, among others by Glover, Gordon et al., Haenszel; in Great Britain, among others by McKenzie et al., Stocks, Case, Kennaway, Ashley; in Switzerland, by Schinz and Reich; in Denmark, by Clemmesen; in Australia, by Lancaster. Mortality rate compendia are published by the World Health Organization [124] and by Segi et al. [161]. Information on cancer incidence is more limited because it is available only for smaller populations, of the size of a few millions at most — like Scandinavian countries, Connecticut, or selected regions of Poland. Incidence data, with some characteristics of the registries which produced them, have been compiled by Doll et al. [41].

In spite of all the differences listed above, the information derived from mortality statistics and from morbidity registration is not contradictory, but com-

---

* Denmark, England, Finland, France, Norway, United States.

plementary: experience shows that conclusions based on both these sources of information coincide to a large extent.

It has been demonstrated that accuracy in determining the cause of death is higher for cancer than for other diseases [71,123].

2.6. Selection of the Basis of Evaluation of Cancer Occurrence in Poland

In analyzing cancer occurrence in Poland, we shall base our observations mainly on mortality statistics, because:

1. In the four selected regions described in Chapter 2.2, the improvement of cancer reporting and registration first started about 1964. Hence, the incidence data obtained are not yet suitable for the analysis of time trends.

2. Polish cancer incidence data do not depict well the cancer geography of the country as a whole because of large regional variation in the completness of cancer reporting and because of inaccuracies in registration occurring outside of the registries in the four selected regions.

3. Comparison with the cancer risk of Polish migrants is possible only for mortality data because comparable incidence data are not available. Comparison of cancer occurrence in Poland with occurrence in other countries is also easier when based on mortality statistics concerning each country as a whole than it would be if based on data from cancer registration in selected regions of those countries, because selection of such regions and their representativeness for the respective countries varies and is difficult to evaluate. However, information from mortality statistics will be compared, whenever possible, with incidence data from cancer registries.

2.7. Scope of the Present Study

Following a discussion of all cancer sites * combined, subsequent chapters will deal with cancer of the stomach, intestinal tract, lung, uterus, breast and prostate, which are the most frequent and socially most important cancers; altogether they are responsible for 60 percent of cancer deaths in Poland. Their common features are a low proportion of nonepithelial tumors (as may be seen in Appendix Table 21), their infrequent occurrence in childhood and adolescence, and their increasing occurrence with advancing age.

---

* "Site" as used here and throughout this monograph refers specifically to an organ or part of the body subject to cancer.

3*

Cancer of the liver, biliary passages, or pancreas will not be considered because their diagnosis is the least accurate. Skin cancer is omitted because of the low fatality rate which largely decreases the value of mortality statistics as estimates of its occurrence. Other cancer sites are also not considered since their lower incidence indicates both their lesser social importance and the fact that conclusions based upon data about them would be vague.

3 | Methods

Age is one of the most important factors related to cancer risk and must be considered in all comparisons of data on cancer occurrence.

3.1. Graphic Comparisons

The semi-log scale, presenting age on the arithmetic and cancer incidence or mortality on the logarithmic axis, will be used for most of the graphic comparisons. Most cancers are characterized by an approximately constant rate of risk increase with age, at least in some age interval. In the semi-log scale a constant rate of change is presented as a straight line relationship — therefore, this scale depicts the rate of change better than the usual, arithmetic scale. An additional advantage of the semi-log scale is that it presents relations well when one of the variables shows a wide range, e.g.: from 0.1 to 100.0, as is usual with mortality rates by age.

In accordance with a common, if not quite formally correct practice, the last, open age group "85 and over" will be presented in the graphs as if it were 85–89 *. On the graphs depicting cancer incidence, the last, open age groups will not be shown because they are too large, and of a varying extent: 60 and over for the Warszawa registry, and 70 and over for the three other registries.

In interpreting the graphs, general tendencies should be considered rather than the individual rates, which may have a large random variation if based on small numbers. This concerns especially the mortality rates of migrants to Australia and, to a lesser extent, the incidence rates for rural areas (for all cancer sites combined the number of deaths or new cases, from which these rates were computed was, respectively, 460 and 1638), and for younger age groups.

The age groups below 25—30 will not usually be presented on the graphs because of the relative rarity of cancer in this period of life, resulting in large random variation, as well as because of its different character: nonepithelial neoplasms predominate in these young age groups.

---

* In the case of the 1950 mortality rates for Polish-born Americans, the open age group "75 and over" is depicted in the graphs as 80 years.

3.2. Mortality and Incidence Rates, Standardization

The frequency of cancer occurrence (its risk or probability) can be estimated from either morbidity or mortality data. From morbidity data, usually derived from cancer registration, **cancer incidence** can be determined: the probability, in a given population, of an individual contracting the disease in question within a unit of time. It is measured by the **incidence rate**, computed by dividing the number of new cases of cancer observed in a given population in the period of a year by the number of that population. The result is usually multiplied by 100,000 to avoid fractions; a rate per 100,000 of the specified population is thus obtained.

In an analogous manner, **cancer mortality** or the probability in a given population of death from the disease in question is ascertained from mortality statistics. It is measured by the **mortality rate.** This rate is, by analogy, a ratio of the deaths registered for that disease in one year to the population in which they were registered. Mortality differs thus from **fatality,** which is the risk of people with the disease to die from it.

The **age-specific rates** will be used, when possible, computed for either 5- or 10-year age groups. They illustrate best the risk of cancer. These rates are presented in Appendix Tables 3-16 and in most of the graphs. The actual observed numbers, from which any of the rates was computed, can be calculated easily from these tables: the rate in question, divided by the "rate per case" shown in the table for the respective sex- and age-group, gives the observed number of new cancer cases or deaths, approximate because of rounding off.

For international comparisons, as well as for analysis of regional data, comparison of dozens of sets of age-specific rates would be too unwieldy. In such cases **summarizing indices** have to be used. **Only age-adjusted (age-standardized) rates** will be used, since the crude rates would be useless because of the wide differences of the age structure of the populations compared. For example, the crude 1959–61 cancer mortality rate was five times higher in Polish-born American females than in Poland, whereas the age-adjusted rate was only 62 percent higher. Age-adjustment corrects here for the big difference in the age-structure of the populations compared. For example 60 percent of the population of Poland was below the age of 35, compared with only five percent of Polish migrants.

Age-adjusted rates have generally been computed by the **direct method** [76,166]. For international comparisons, the "world population" proposed by Segi et al. [160,161], usually as modified by Doll et al. [41], will be used as the standard. Finding that the results obtained when using either of them differed only by about 0.5 percent, we feel that comparison of standardized rates based on either one of both forms of standard is permissible, since the possible distortion of results is negligible.

The 95 percent confidence limits of the age-adjusted rates, presented in Appendix Table 17, are computed using the formula given by Spiegelman [166]:

$$\text{standard deviation} = \sqrt{\sum w_x^2 \cdot \frac{D_x}{P_x^2}}$$

where w_x is the weight ascribed to the age group x by the standard used, i.e. the proportion of that age group in the standard population;

D_x — number of deaths in the age group x;

P_x — number of persons in that age group;

$\left(\dfrac{D_x}{P_x}\right)$ is thus the age-specific rate in the age-group x.

As can be seen from Appendix Table 17, confidence limits are not necessary for the interpretation of data on Poland or on native white Americans, both of which have a small variation coefficient. On the other hand, rates for Polish migrants are based on much smaller numbers of deaths so that the confidence limits are often quite broad.

Because not only are the accuracy and reliability of cancer mortality data lower in the oldest age groups, but also their comparability, the age-adjusted rates computed by the direct method will be presented in a way which shows their two components: below and over the age of 65. These components are called **"age--adjusted indexes"**. They are computed by multiplying the age-specific rates by the respective fractions of the total standard population, followed by summing up the results through two ranges of age: 0–64, and 65 and over. Justification of these indexes is given in my work from 1969 [175].

3.3. Regional Differences

For regional comparisons within Poland, the structure of the total 1960 census population (presented in Appendix Table 1) has been used as the standard [18]. Only for 1961 could we compute the age-specific rates by district. These have been published for some cancer sites [170,172,173,184].

For the later period, 1967–69, comparison of cancer mortality by region by the direct method of adjustment was impossible, since no age-specific rates could be computed by district of residence. Hence, the **indirect method** of adjustment was used. For each district the expected number of deaths was computed for every age group by multiplying its population by the standard, which was the age-specific mortality rate for the corresponding age, sex and period in Poland, as shown in Appendix Table 7. The sum of expected deaths in all age groups was used to divide the observed number of deaths in the same district and period. The result, multiplied by 100, is the **standardized mortality ratio SMR** [76]. The SMR's for 1967–69 are presented in Appendix Table 18 along with confidence limits, computed using the tabular values of 95 percent confidence limit factors for estimates of a Poisson-distributed variable from [67]. These SMR's are also presented on maps located among figures in the text of the chapters from four to ten.

In computing the SMR's, five-year age groups were used, terminating at 70 and over because, regretably, no breakdown of the age group over 70 was available for that period *. This is unfortunate because a large part of cancer deaths falls into that age group, the regional variations in the structure of which are not known and cannot be allowed for. This lowers the accuracy of SMR as a measure of regional cancer occurrence — to a lesser extent for cancers such as breast or uterine cancer, the risk of which does not change much after the age of 70, but seriously for prostate cancer, the risk of which rapidly increases with age.

3.4. U/R and M/F Ratios

In comparing cancer mortality in urban and rural populations, the urban-rural ratio of mortality rates, U/R, will be presented. It was computed by dividing the urban rates by the rural ones, using either the age-adjusted (never the crude) rates, or the age-specific rates when the U/R ratios by age are compared.

Presenting the relation between cancer occurrence and sex, the sex ratio of mortality rates, M/F, will be used. It was computed by dividing either the age--adjusted or the age-specific male mortality rates by the corresponding female rates.

For incidence data neither the age-specific sex ratios nor the urban-rural ones will be discussed because of the large inherent random variation.

* The respective population data, derived from a study of the age- and sex-structure of the population as of December 31, 1967 [219], are presented in Appendix Table 19.

4 | Cancer-All Sites*

4 1 Opening Remarks

According to the Polish mortality statistics, cancer accounted for 17 percent of all deaths in 1969, an increase from 9.5 percent in 1959. This increase can be ascribed to an increase in longevity in Poland, because frequency of cancer occurrence increases with age; to a decreasing mortality from some other diseases, especially the infectious ones; to improved diagnosis; and to a true increase in the frequency of occurrence of some types of cancer.

4.2. Poland and Other Countries

Compared with mortality rates in 24 countries in 1964–65, Poland ranks next after white Americans: 18th for males and 20th for females (Figures 4-1 and 4-2). Polish incidence rates for cancer of all sites combined belong among the low ones in comparison with other countries [41].

4.3. Sex

Mortality rates from cancer of all sites combined are higher for Polish males than for females. The M/F ratio increased from 1.30 : 1 in 1959–61 to 1.42 : 1 in 1967–69. This increase occurred in all age groups (Figure 4-3). As in other countries, it was a result of the increase in male lung cancer mortality.

For most age groups the M/F ratio equals approximately 1.5 : 1, but during the ages 30–50 the high proportion of cancer of the uterine cervix and of the breast leads to an excess of female over male mortality.

An excess of male over female mortality for cancer of all sites combined is observed in all 24 countries for which cancer mortality data are published by Segi

---

* Sites of cancer included are Numbers 140–205, *International Classification of Diseases*, 1955 revision.

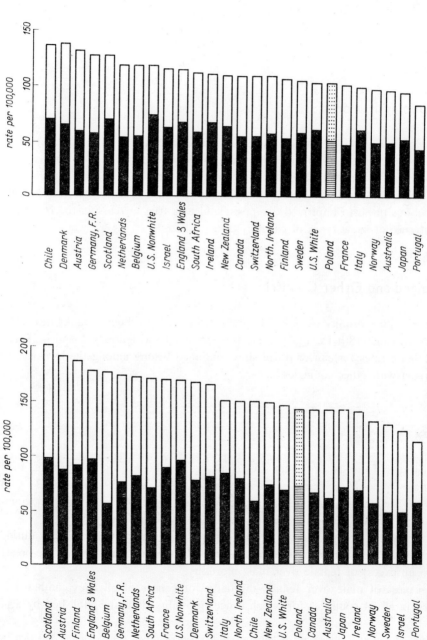

Fig. 4-1. Age-adjusted mortality rates for cancer, all sites combined (Nos. 140–205, *ICD,* 1955 rev.), per 100,000 males in 1964–65 in 24 countries [161] and in Poland.

Fig. 4-2. Age-adjusted mortality rates for cancer, all sites combined (Nos. 140–205, *ICD,* 1955 rev.), per 100,000 females in 1964–65 in 24 countries [161] and in Poland.

Remark to Fig. 4-1 and 4-2. Shaded areas represent mortality under the age of 65.

et al. [161]. In 1964–65 the M/F ratio was lowest in Israel (1.02 : 1), but exceeded 1.5 : 1 in Finland, Great Britain and France. In the past few years it has displayed an upward trend in all these countries.

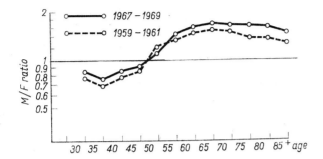

Fig. 4-3. Male/female ratios, M/F, of the age-specific mortality rates for cancer, all sites combined (Nos. 140–205, *ICD*, 1955 rev.), in 1959–61 and 1967–69 in Poland.

4.4. Age

As a rule the frequency of cancer occurrence increases from the age of about 15–20 up to the oldest age groups. The slowing-down of that increase among the oldest age-groups, causing a downturn of the mortality-by-age curve (Figures 4-4 and 4-5) is, however, characteristic of Poland. This phenomenon was more conspicuous in 1959–61 than in 1967–69 and more for rural than for urban population.

A similar downturn of the mortality-by-age curve could be noticed in 1958–59 in Japan and in nonwhite Americans; in 1964–65 it was less conspicuous. It was absent from the data of the other of the 24 countries reported by Segi et al. [160,161], which, however, did not show a breakdown of the age group 75 and over for Portugal or 65 and over for Chile.

When the cancer mortality-by-age curves in selected regions of Poland in 1961 are compared, the largest differences in their shape are noticeable in oldest age groups. Whereas only a slight slowing-down of the speed of cancer mortality increase with age is observed for the five metropolitan cities, in other regions, most conspicuously in the eastern districts, mortality rates decrease after the age of 70–75. The regional cancer mortality differences are thus more conspicuous at ages over 70 (Figure 4-6).

Data from cancer registration in the four selected regions indicate that up to the age of 60 also the cancer incidence is similar in all these regions (Figures 4-7 and

4-8) except for females in Warszawa City where the rates for all the age groups are higher than in other regions (a situation that can only partly be accounted for by the inclusion of the in situ cervix uteri carcinoma — see Chapter 9.1). Analysis

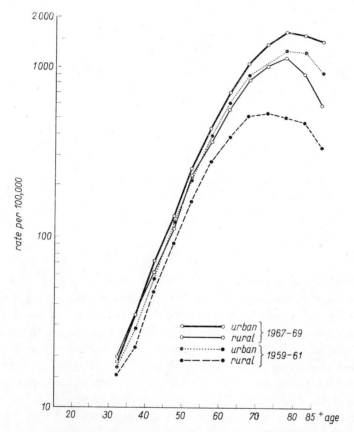

Fig. 4-4. Age-specific mortality rates for cancer, all sites combined (Nos. 140–205, *ICD*, 1955 rev.), per 100,000 males, by urban-rural residence in 1959–61 and 1967–69 in Poland.

of cancer incidence in older age groups is impossible because their detailed age structure is unknown; such analysis should be possible after publication of the results of the 1970 census.

4.5. Residence

Cancer mortality for all sites combined is higher for the urban than for the rural population in Poland. This excess of urban over rural mortality rates includes all age groups (Figures 4-4, 4-5, 4-9, 4-10), but the older to a higher degree than the

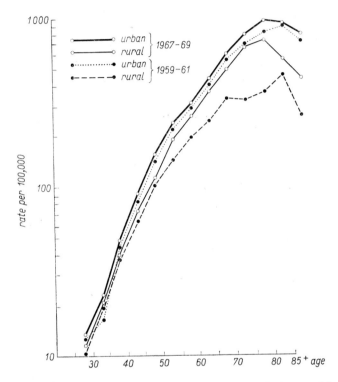

Fig. 4-5. Age-specific mortality rates for cancer, all sites combined (Nos. 140–205, *ICD*, 1955 rev.), per 100,000 females, by urban-rural residence in 1959–61 and 1967–69 in Poland.

younger ones. The urban-rural ratio, U/R, for males decreased from 1.62 : 1 in 1959–61 to 1.27 : 1 in 1967–69, and for females from 1.65 : 1 to 1.23 : 1 in the same period. This decrease was larger for the older than for the younger age-

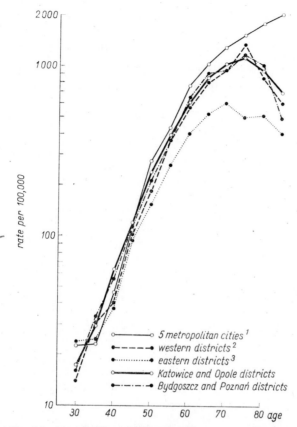

Fig. 4-6. Age-specific mortality rates for cancer, all sites combined (Nos. 140–205, *ICD*, 1955 rev.), per 100,000 males, in 1961 in the selected regions of Poland. 1 — Warszawa, Kraków, Łódź, Poznań and Wrocław City, 2 — Szczecin, Koszalin, Zielona Góra and Wrocław District, 3 — Białystok, Lublin and Rzeszów District.

-groups. Polish cancer registration data also indicate a cancer incidence higher in urban than in rural populations [88],[98],[99],[100]. Occurrence of cancer more frequently in urban than in rural populations was noted in other countries too. For example, the U/R ratio in Norway was 1.35 : 1 for males and 1.20 : 1 for females [41].

Data on regional differences in age-adjusted cancer mortality rates in 1961 in Poland were presented in a previous paper [170]. The highest mortality rates for all cancer sites combined were observed in 5 metropolitan cities, and the lowest ones in the eastern districts. In 1967–69 the ranking of the districts remained relatively unchanged, but the range between rates for the metropolitan cities and the eastern districts diminished from 2 : 1 to 1.5 : 1. The SMR's for 1967–69 are presented in Appendix Table 18 and in Figures 4-11 and 4-12.

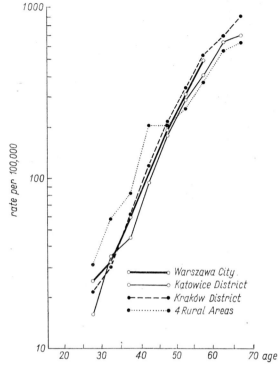

Fig. 4-7. Age-specific incidence rates for cancer, all sites combined (Nos. 140–205, *ICD*, 1955 rev.), per 100,000 males in 1965–66 in the four regions of Poland.

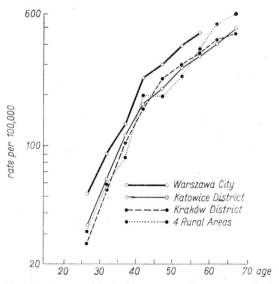

Fig. 4-8. Age-specific incidence rates for cancer, all sites combined (Nos. 140–205, *ICD*, 1955 rev.), per 100,000 females in 1965–66 in the four regions of Poland.

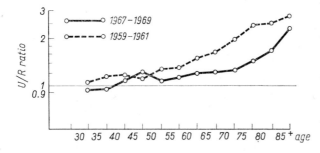

Fig. 4–9. Urban-rural ratios, *U/R*, of the age-specific mortality rates for cancer, all sites combined (Nos. 140–205, *ICD*, 1955 rev.), for males in 1959–61 and 1967–69 in Poland.

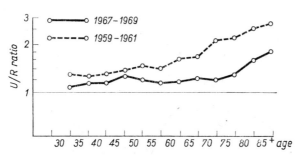

Fig. 4–10. Urban-rural ratios, *U/R*, of the age-specific mortality rates for cancer, all sites combined (Nos. 140–205, *ICD*, 1955 rev.), for females in 1959–61 and 1967–69 in Poland.

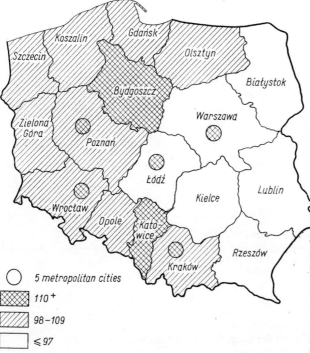

Fig. 4-11. Standardized mortality ratios, SMR, for cancer, all sites combined (Nos. 140–205, *ICD*, 1955 rev.), for males by district of residence in 1967–69 in Poland. SMR = 100 for the total Polish population of the same sex and in the same period.

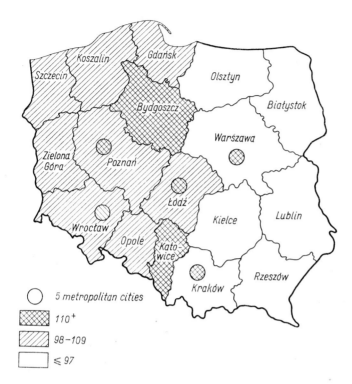

Fig. 4-12. Standardized mortality ratios, SMR, for cancer, all sites combined (Nos. 140–205, *ICD*, 1955 rev.), for females by district of residence in 1967–69 in Poland. SMR = 100 for the total Polish population of the same sex and in the same period.

4.6. Time Trends

Information on cancer occurrence in Poland prior to 1959 is fragmentary. Only the three most important sources will be discussed.

Krasuska [102] described cancer mortality statistics for Warszawa City for 1882–1963. Throughout most of that period all deaths were certified by physicians. Between 1921–1931 a distinct cancer mortality increase was noted only for the over 60 age group. In the 1921–1960 period the crude mortality rates per 100,000 population increased from 43 to 68 for cancer of the alimentary tract, from 8 to 25 for cancer of the breast or genital organs, and from 4 (in 1931) to 23 for cancer of the respiratory tract.

Bielecki and Piekutowska [17] compared cancer mortality in Warszawa City in 1889–1892 and 1951–55 and found that it increased only for individuals over the age of 60, an increase accompanied by a decrease in the rate of deaths certified due to senility. They also analyzed cancer occurrence in Poland on the basis of the

1949–1955 mortality and 1951–1955 morbidity. Among other things they conclude: "Differences in (cancer) mortality between Poland and other countries depend on the different age structure of the population and on the poorer diagnosis of this cause of death, especially in the older age groups. Diagnostic mistakes are the main cause of the apparant lower rural mortality".

The autopsy series of the Jagiellonian University Pathologic Institute in Kraków, published for 1851–1938 by Ciechanowski [28] and for 1939–1958 by Kulig et al. [105] is one of the world's largest. In this material, cancer of the stomach is seen to be first in rank in both time series. Further, a decrease by half of the proportion of stomach cancer found during autopsies is apparent over the last 70 years, as is a 10-fold increase of lung cancer. Also increasing was the proportion of autopsies where laryngeal and urinary bladder cancer were found, whereas a decrease for esophageal and lip cancer was noted. Autopsy statistics, however, like hospital statistics, are not reliable sources of data on cancer occurrence in a population. The autopsy data mentioned, therefore, are not sufficient to tell without doubt if the risk of stomach cancer truly decreased. It may be that the proportion decreased because of an increase in the frequency of other cancers, together with changes in the selection of people being admitted to hospitals and subjected to postmortem examinations upon death. On the other hand, the increase in the proportion of lung cancer was so large that it points to a true increase in lung cancer risk in Poland.

Returning to cancer mortality for the whole of Poland, we observe a distinct increase in the rates for both sexes between 1959 and 1969. As shown in Figures

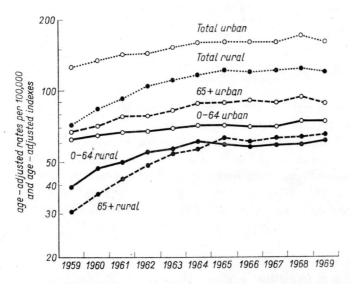

Fig. 4-13. Time trends in age-adjusted mortality rates and "age-adjusted indexes" up to and over 65 years of age, for cancer, all sites combined (Nos. 140–205, *ICD,* 1955 rev.), for males by urban-rural residence in the 1959–1969 period in Poland.

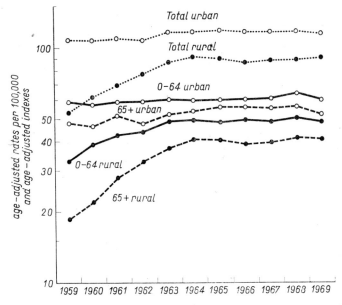

Fig. 4-14. Time trends in age-adjusted mortality rates and "age-adjusted indexes" up to and over 65 years of age, for cancer, all sites combined (Nos. 140–205, *ICD*, 1955 rev.), for females by urban-rural residence in the 1959–1969 period in Poland.

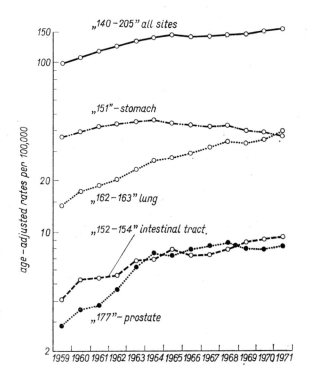

Fig. 4-15. Time trends in age--adjusted mortality rates for cancer of all sites combined and of selected sites, per 100,000 males in the 1959–1971 period in Poland.

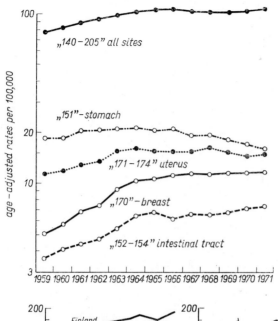

Fig. 4–16. Time trends in age--adjusted mortality rates for cancer of all sites combined and of selected sites, per 100,000 females in the 1959–1971 period in Poland.

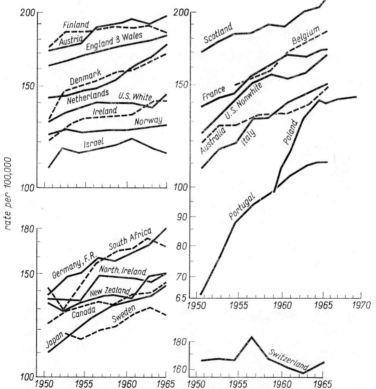

Fig. 4-17. Time trends in age-adjusted mortality rates for cancer, all sites combined (Nos. 140–205, *ICD*, 1955 rev.), per 100,000 males in the 1950–1965 period as reported by Segi et al. [160,161], and in the 1959–1969 period in Poland.

4-13, 4-14, 4-15, and 4-16, the increase continued until about 1963 and stopped almost completely thereafter. This increase in cancer mortality was more marked in the rural than in the urban population and greater among the older than among the younger age groups. It was most distinct in the eastern districts and least in the metropolitan cities. The slowing down in the increase of cancer mortality around 1963 was also most marked in rural populations and in older age groups.

Mortality for some of the major sites (discussed in more detail in subsequent chapters) is also shown in Figures 4-15 and 4-16. The greatest increases evident are those in lung cancer among males and breast cancer among females. Although stomach cancer mortality initially increased, it afterwards showed a tendency to decrease.

The increase of cancer in Poland was, especially for females, more rapid than the increase in the 24 countries for which mortality data has been compiled by Segi et al. [160,161]. In the 1950–1965 period the cancer mortality rate for males increased in all of these countries except Switzerland; but for females it increased distinctly only in Portugal, decreased in a few countries, and remained constant in most (Figures 4-17 and 4-18).

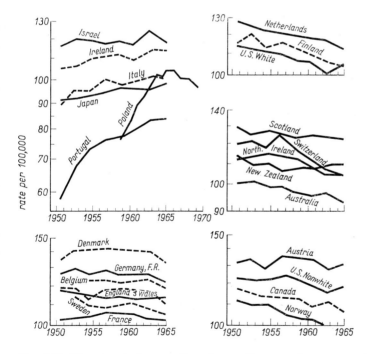

Fig. 4-18. Time trends in age-adjusted mortality rates for cancer, all sites combined (Nos. 140–205, *ICD*, 1955 rev.), per 100,000 females in the 1950–1965 period as reported by Segi et al. [160,161], and in the 1959–1969 period in Poland.

4.7. Polish Migrants

The decrease, in the oldest age groups, of cancer mortality with advancing age was absent among Polish migrants to the United States and Australia (Figures 4-19 and 4-20).

In the United States, between 1950 and 1959–61, mortality from cancer, all sites, among Polish migrants has increased for the older age groups, especially males, whereas it decreased for the younger ones: for females under 55 and for males under 65. Notwithstanding, cancer mortality rates among Polish-born Americans in 1959–61 were higher than they were in Poland or among native white Americans for each age group except males under 55.

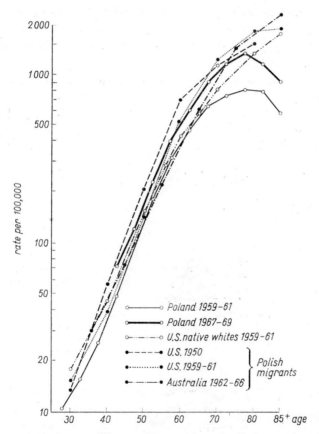

Fig. 4-19. Age-specific mortality rates for cancer, all sites combined (Nos. 140–205, *ICD*, 1955 rev.), per 100,000 males, in Poland, in Polish migrants to the United States and to Australia, and in native white Americans.

Between 1950 and 1959–61 age-adjusted cancer mortality rates among native white Americans increased by 7 percent for males and decreased by the same amount for females, whereas among Polish-born Americans they decreased by 5 percent for males and did not change for females.

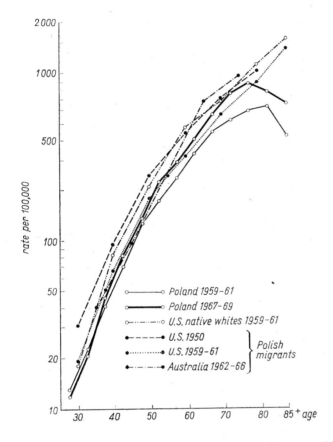

Fig. 4-20. Age-specific mortality rates for cancer, all sites combined (Nos. 140–205, *ICD*, 1955 rev.), per 100,000 females, in Poland, in Polish migrants to the United States and to Australia, and in native white Americans.

4.8. Discussion

Cancer is not a single disease but a group of diseases (differing — often to a large extent — in their course, prognosis, and epidemiologic characteristics) all of which should be analyzed separately. These diseases are usually classified according to the primary sites — to the organs primarily involved. It should be remembered, however, that quite different cancers may develop in the same organ. The cancer chapter of the *International Classification of Diseases* makes some distinctions but not always completely. For instance, adenocarcinoma of the uterine corpus and squamous cell carcinoma of the uterine cervix are sometimes distinguished, but often combined as "uterus, unspecified". More frequently, this classification combines various cancers developing in the same organ into one class. For example, carcinoma of the kidney, occurring in adults as a rule, and Wilms' tumor, frequent in childhood but exceptional in adults, are considered jointly as "cancer of the kidney".

The main purpose of the following discussion of all cancers combined is to determine the most general characteristics of data on their occurrence in Poland, to find their relation to age, sex and residence, and to create a background for more detailed analyses of data on cancer of particular sites.

4.8.1. Sex

In Poland, as in other countries, the risk of most cancers is higher among males than among females. This sex differential is most pronounced for respiratory and upper alimentary tract cancers. Cancers of the breast, of the genitals, of the thyroid, or of the biliary passages are more frequent in females.

The more frequent occurrence of cancer among males can be explained partly by environmental or social factors, such as occupational hazards or tobacco smoking. Even in childhood and adolescence, however, males are subject to a higher cancer risk than females. This relationship between cancer risk and sex may be due to hormonal and metabolic differences which, for example, may indirectly modify the action of chemical carcinogens by their effect on cell membrane permeability: estrogenic and androgenic hormones significantly control the entry of particulate matter into cells in experimental models [101]. It has also been suggested that, because they possess the double X chromosome, females have a higher immunologic potential which helps to destroy incipient neoplastic cells and thus decreases the frequency of overt clinical tumors [11]. One of the possible tests of this hypothesis might be to determine the frequency of cancer occurrence among males with the Klinefelter syndrome, possessing double X chromosome.

4.8.2. Age

With cancer of most sites, as with carcinomas of the alimentary tract, skin, or prostate, the relation between risk and age can be approximated by the exponential or power function, and is thus approximately linear when plotted on the semi-log or log-log scale (logarithm of risk against either age or logarithm of age).

These scales also generate other shapes of the risk-by-age curve:

1. A risk peak in childhood followed by a decline, as is the case with Wilms' tumor.

2. A peak in later life exemplified by lung cancer in males.

3. An age-risk curve consisting of two linear segments, the first having a steeper slope than the second, exemplified by breast or cervix uteri cancer.

4. Two peaks as is the case with Hodgkin's disease.

Doll presents an interesting discussion of the significance and shape of cancer age-risk relationships and curves [38]. It may be assumed that for epithelial cancers of most sites the risk I, as measured by incidence or mortality, increases proportionally to the kth power of age:

$$I = b \cdot t^k$$

where t is age, b is a constant.

Doll observed that for each cancer site the values of k are similar in various populations, whereas b may differ much, but they differ for various cancer sites, ranging from about 4 for skin to 11 for prostate. For lung cancer among smokers k equals about 7.5, and about 4 among nonsmokers.

If, in the above equation, age is replaced by the length of exposure to the carcinogenic factor $t - w$, where w is the sum of the time before exposure plus the preclinical cancer development, assumed by Doll as 2.5 years, the equation becomes

$$I = b(t - w)^k$$

Then for lung cancer for both nonsmokers (for whom exposure since birth is assumed) and for smokers, k becomes about 4 and b is proportional to the average daily dose of the carcinogenic factor, in this case to the daily number of cigarettes smoked.

Doll deduces that continuous exposure to a carcinogenic factor results in a power function relation between age and cancer incidence (straight line on a log-log diagram) and that an unusually rapid increase in cancer risk with age is due either to a long pre-exposure or pre-clinical period or to a reduction in the exposure of successive cohorts * to the environmental carcinogens. Increasing exposure of successive cohorts, conversely, leads to a slowing of the rate of risk increase with age among the older age-groups as is the case with lung cancer in males. A decreased rate of increase of risk after some age, as with breast or cervix uteri cancer, or as with lung cancer among those who stopped smoking, indicates a reduction in or cessation of exposure to carcinogenic factors. A peak of risk in childhood or early adolescence may be due to a brief exposure to a carcinogenic factor or to increased mitotic activity.

* A cohort is defined as a group of persons born in the same period (year, 5 years, etc.). Cohort analysis of cancer risk requires data from a longer period than available in our material.

In the case of bimodal curves, it is assumed that they may either be caused by the action of different factors in various periods of life or by the fact that a disease may be not just one but two or more different cancers, as MacMahon has postulated for Hodgkin's disease [113].

Little is known yet on the relation between the effect of a carcinogenic factor and the age at which it acts. It seems that such relationships may vary for different carcinogens and for different cancers.

Also related to age is the accuracy and comparability of information on cancer occurrence; both decrease for the oldest age groups [30,37,170].

The cessation of the increase in cancer mortality with advancing age observed in Poland in the oldest age groups was probably a spurious phenomenon, the result of less accuracy of cancer diagnosis and death certification in these age groups. Such a conclusion is supported by the absence of this phenomenon from the 1961 mortality rates for metropolitan cities (Figure 4-6), where the quality of mortality statistics was best, as well as by the partial disappearance of this phenomenon for other regions of Poland in recent years. The fact that this abnormality in the mortality-to-age relation does not occur among Polish migrants also points in the same direction; the only alternative would be the existence of some factor operative in Poland, but not characteristic of the Polish population. This same phenomenon is also disappearing in populations such as Japan where it appeared not long ago.

4.8.3. Residence and Time Trends

Cancer mortality in Poland is lower among rural than among urban populations. The range between urban and rural mortality rates decreased in the 1959–1969 period, especially for the older age groups; and the range between the highest rates, reported for the metropolitan cities, and the lowest rates, for eastern districts, diminished.

What is the reason for these changes and for the regional differences? Two explanations suggest themselves:

1. Differences and changes in exposure to carcinogenic factors. There are differences between the habits, customs and environment of urban and rural populations. Also the districts where cancer mortality rates are lowest differ from the other districts with respect to these factors. These differences have been decreasing in recent years so that corresponding changes in exposure to carcinogenic factors, which might lead to observable differences and changes in cancer risks, seem quite probable. Such an explanation is further supported by the prevalence of urban over rural cancer risk observed in other countries. Comparisons and interpretations, however, are difficult because "the definitions of urban and rural areas are more arbitrary than often realized and vary from one country to another" [29].

2. Regional differences and changes in accuracy of establishing causes of deaths. During the 1959–1969 period the Polish Health Service developed most rapidly in those very regions where it was least developed at the beginning of the period. The transportation system enjoyed the same kind of growth. Appendix Table 20 shows the increase in the number of physicians and hospital beds per 10,000 population and the increase in length of roads per 100 square kilometers. For those regions, in which cancer mortality rates also were initially the lowest and increased most rapidly, presumably the initial level of availability of medical services also was the lowest and increased most rapidly. This conclusion is supported by the tabulation of the proportion of deaths certified by physicians. During the period analysed this proportion increased for rural areas from 45 percent to 85 percent while in urban areas it remained at about 97 percent. In the eastern districts it was lowest but increased most.

Regional differences in the quality of mortality statistics and the decrease in the range of quality between the more and less developed regions is demonstrated by a useful index to the quality of mortality statistics: the proportion of deaths certified as due to "senility, symptoms and other ill-defined conditions" (Nos. 780–795, *ICD*, 1955 revision). Cancer accounts for a substantial, but difficult to evaluate, proportion of that class. Freudenberg estimated that it is the cause of approximately 20–30 percent of deaths certified as the result of senility [51].

The number of deaths classified as the result of senility, symptoms and other ill-defined conditions has markedly decreased, especially in the eastern districts, in spite of the increased proportion of the oldest age groups, among which these causes of death are most frequently diagnosed (Appendix Table 20). Data presented in this table permit us to estimate the trends of changes, but not the regional differences. For the latter purpose the age-adjusted rates are indispensable. Data required for their computation were available only for 1961, and these rates were presented in an earlier paper [170]. As was to be expected, the highest mortality rates ascribed to senility, symptoms and other ill-defined conditions were found in those districts where cancer mortality rates were the lowest.

The increase in reported cancer mortality in Poland was marked before about 1963–1964, but slowed down in later years. This increase was apparently related to the improvement in determinating causes of death. One of the main reasons for this improvement was probably a regulation issued by the Ministry of Health and Welfare on August 3, 1961, introducing the requirement that a death certificate can be issued only by a physician or, in some cases, by his assistant or by a nurse or midwife. It is conceivable that this regulation was fully implemented in one or two years, and that further improvement in the certification of causes of death is a result of increasing professional qualifications of physicians rather than of administrative actions.

4.8.4 Interpretation of Data on Cancer Occurrence
in Poland during 1959-1969

Each of the above explanations for the observed time trends and regional differences in cancer occurrence in Poland may be partly correct. Most of these changes and differences, however, probably depend on the accuracy with which cancer is diagnosed and certified as a cause of death. Such a conclusion is supported not only by the previous discussion, but even more so by another observation: similarities in patterns of occurrence of cancers of various primary sites.

Cancers of all sites were considered jointly in the present chapter. It will be shown in the following chapters, that during the period under consideration, both regional patterns of and time trends in occurrence of cancers of a number of different primary sites were similar; so that it seems unlikely that such similarity could be the result of regional differences or changes in exposure to carcinogenic factors, because such factors differ for various cancers. Some cancers are more frequent in wealthy populations, whereas others occur more frequently among the poor. The risk of some cancers is increased among married, multiparous women, while the risk of others is higher among single, childless women. Some cancers are associated with exposure to sunshine, to X-rays, to certain chemicals, or with nutrition and dietary habits. Hence, it seems unlikely that all such cancers, depending on various, sometimes even opposite factors, could have a similar regional distribution or display simultanous changes in time trends. It is much more likely that the common factor, which produces similarities in both regional patterns and time trends for cancers of various etiopathogenesis, is their detectability.

The further conclusion is evident that not much attention should be given to an increase in Polish cancer mortality rates limited to the oldest age groups (especially in rural populations and in the eastern districts) or to the period prior to 1964; such increase is probably spurious, resulting from improved diagnosis of cancer and its certification as a cause of death. On the other hand, an increase in cancer mortality rates occurring in the age groups under 65 indicates a true increase in cancer risk, especially when it was apparent both in urban populations and after 1964. The relatively low cancer mortality rates in the eastern districts, compared to other districts, as well as the cessation of the mortality increase with age in the oldest age groups, are due to poorer cancer detection and reporting rather than to a lower frequency of cancer occurrence in these districts in respective age-groups.

The incidence data from Polish cancer registries presented here do not permit a similar discussion, because the period of observation is too short for evaluation of time trends, and data on cancer incidence in the oldest age groups are insufficient.

5 | Stomach Cancer

5.1. Opening Remarks

Stomach cancer is the most frequent cause of cancer death in Poland, but its relative position is decreasing — from 35 percent in males and 23 percent in females
in 1959–61 to 28 and 19 percent, respectively, in 1967–69. The incidence data from
the four regional registries in 1965–66 rank stomach cancer first in males and
second, after uterine cervix, in females; only in Warszawa does stomach cancer
rank second to lung cancer in males and third after uterine cervix and breast cancer
in females.

Because of its low curability and the usually short period of time between the
diagnosis of stomach cancer and death, mortality and morbidity statistics are
similar for the occurrence of this neoplasm.

5.2. Poland and Other Countries

Poland is among the countries where stomach cancer risk is high. Had Polish
stomach cancer figures been included in Segi's compilation of mortality rates Poland would have ranked third for males, and fourth for females (Figures 5-1
and 5-2).

Incidence data reported from various centers [41] indicate that in the Japanese
and Colombian registries stomach cancer was distinctly more prevalent than in the
Polish ones. A similar or only slightly higher incidence was reported by registries
in Slovenia, Finland, Hungary, GDR and GFR, Newfoundland, South Africa, and
among the Maoris in New Zealand and Hawaiians and Japanese in Hawaii. A very
high risk for stomach cancer has also been reported in Iceland [62] and in some areas
of the USSR [27,119].

5.3. Sex

Stomach cancer mortality in Poland is higher in males than in females. The over-
all M/F ratio was 2.0 : 1 in 1959–61 and increased somewhat in virtually all age
groups, reaching an average of 2.2 : 1 in 1967–69 (Figure 5-3). The M/F ratio

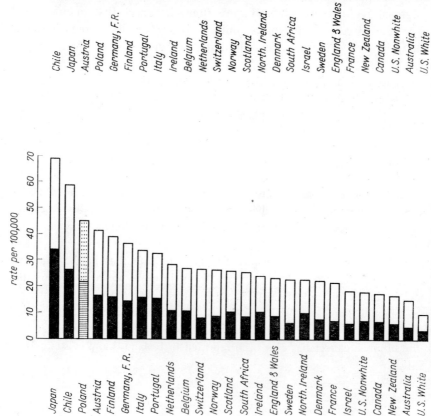

Fig. 5-1. Age-adjusted stomach cancer mortality rates, per 100,000 males, in 1964-65 in 24 countries [161] and in Poland. Shaded areas represent mortality under the age of 65.

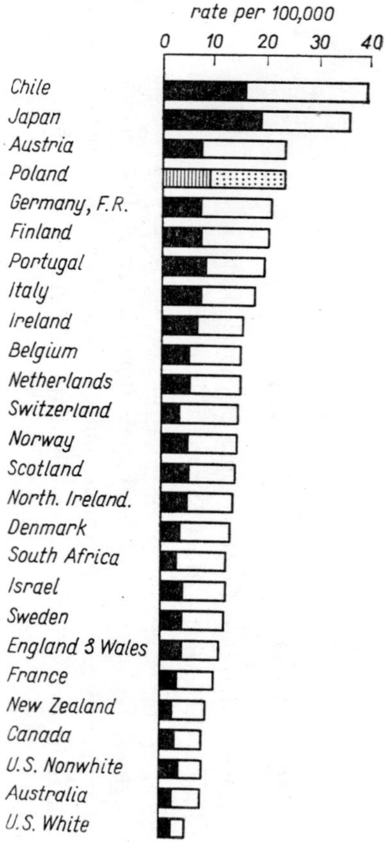

Fig. 5-2. Age-adjusted stomach cancer mortality rates, per 100,000 females, in 1964-65 in 24 countries [161] and in Poland. Shaded areas represent mortality under the age of 65.

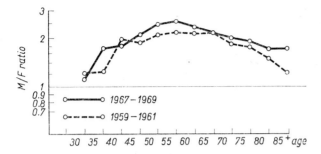

Fig. 5-3. Male/female ratios, M/F, of the age-specific stomach cancer mortality rates, in 1959–61 and 1967–69 in Poland.

observed in Poland may be considered high. In only two out of 24 countries (Canada, United States nonwhites) was the M/F mortality ratio greater than 2.0 : 1 in both 1962–63 and 1964–65. The lowest value, 1.5 : 1, was observed in Israel [160,161]; hence, the range was relatively small.

The M/F ratio in Poland increases with age from about 1.3 : 1 in the 30–34 age group to a maximum value of about 2.5 : 1 at 50–54, decreasing in the older age groups. The same situation was observed in the United States by Gordon et al. [53]. Griffith [57] noticed that this phenomenon is not observed with respect to cancer of other parts of the alimentary tract, but appears in data concerning both stomach cancer mortality and incidence and seems to be constant whether risk is high or low. For both Poland and for native white Americans the M/F ratio-by-age curves for 1959–61 are very similar, despite the fact that mortality rates for this cancer are over four times as high in Poland as in the United States.

5.4. Age

As a rule, stomach cancer risk increases with age up to the oldest age groups [37]. The decrease of the stomach cancer mortality at about the age of 70 years observed in Poland in both males and females was due most probably to incorrect certification of death in the oldest groups, as discussed in Chapter 4 (See Figures 5-4 and 5-5). This decrease in 1967–69 was less distinct than in 1961, especially in the rural population.

Disregarding the oldest age groups, the slope of the age curve in Poland was similar to that in other countries, but in each age group, mortality in Poland was relatively high. The same observation also pertains to incidence.

The rate of increase of stomach cancer risk related to age is slightly higher for males than for females up to about 55 years of age, but lower in the older age groups, resulting in the age-dependent changes in the M/F ratio described in the previous subchapter.

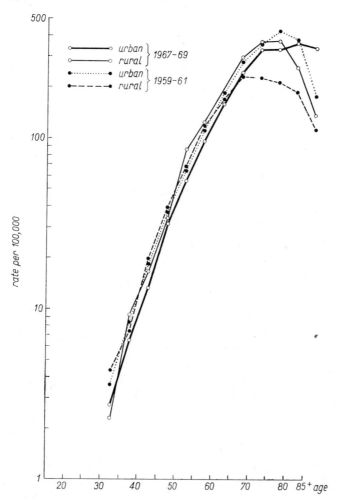

Fig. 5-4. Age-specific stomach cancer mortality rates, per 100,000 males, by urban-rural residence in 1959–61 and 1967–69 in Poland.

5.5. Residence

Unlike other cancers, stomach cancer is responsible for higher mortality in rural than in urban populations in Poland. The U/R ratio changed from 1.21 : 1 in 1959–61 to 0.85 : 1 in 1967–69; it decreased in almost all age groups both for males and females (Figures 5-6 and 5-7).

In 1965–66 stomach cancer incidence under the age 60 was highest in rural areas, intermediate in the mixed ones, and lowest in the city of Warszawa for both males and females (Figures 5-8 and 5-9, Appendix Tables 3-6). Moreover, in the Kraków Region in 1965–68 the incidence of this cancer was higher in rural populations than in the city of Kraków [88].

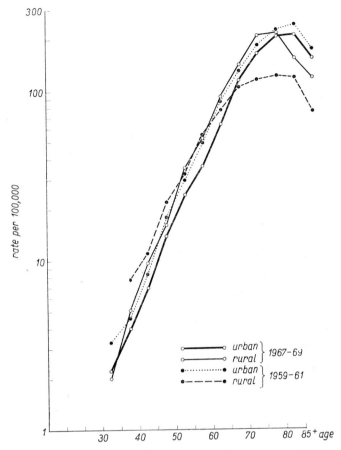

Fig. 5-5. Age-specific stomach cancer mortality rates, per 100,000 females, by urban-rural residence in 1959–61 and 1967–69 in Poland.

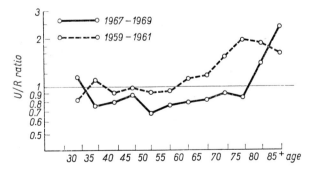

Fig. 5-6. Urban-rural ratios, U/R, of the age-specific stomach cancer mortality rates, for males in 1959–61 and 1967–69 in Poland.

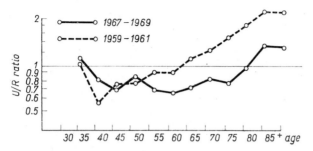

Fig. 5-7. Urban-rural ratios, U/R, of the age-specific stomach cancer mortality rates for females in 1959–61 and 1967–69 in Poland.

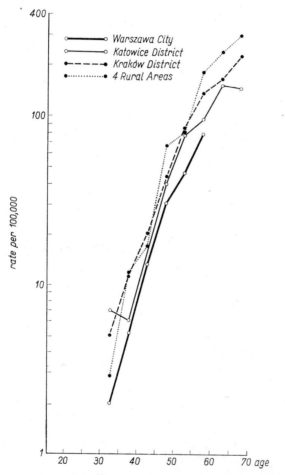

Fig. 5-8. Age-specific stomach cancer incidence rates, per 100,000 males, in 1965–66 in the four regions of Poland.

Stomach cancer incidence was shown to be somewhat lower in rural than in urban populations of Austria and Denmark, whereas in other Scandinavian countries and in the United States the urban-rural differences were insignificant [29,53]. In Czechoslovakia the lowest mortality was observed in Prague; the range between the highest and lowest regional rates was 36 percent [198].

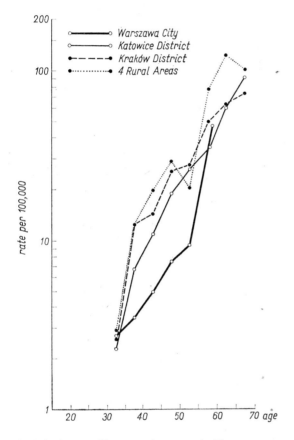

Fig. 5-9. Age-specific stomach cancer incidence rates, per 100,000 females, in 1965–66 in the four regions of Poland.

In Poland regional differences for stomach cancer mortality are less marked than for other cancers. In 1961 the lowest rates were observed in the eastern districts, of which in 1967–69 only Lublin district occupied the same low rank (Figures 5-10 and 5-11, Appendix Table 18). Presently, a low mortality could be observed, for both sexes, in the metropolitan cities which descended markedly in rank compared to 1961.

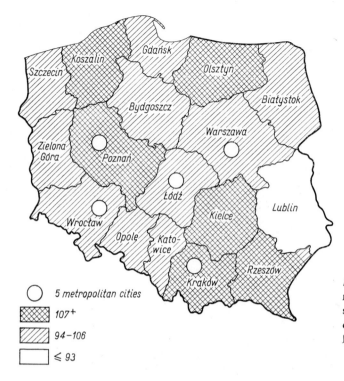

Fig. 5-10. Standardized mortality ratios, SMR, for stomach cancer, by district of residence in 1967–69 in Poland. Males.

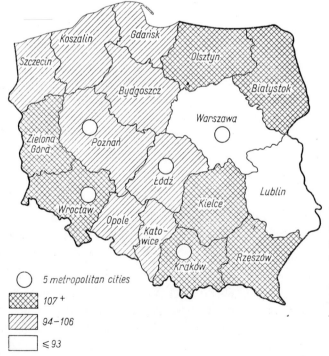

Fig. 5-11. Standardized mortality ratios, SMR, for stomach cancer, by district of residence in 1967–69 in Poland. Females.
SMR = 100 for the total Polish population of the same sex and in the same period.

5.6. Time Trends

Age-adjusted stomach cancer mortality rates increased in Poland in the 1959–1964 period but later decreased. The increase was most marked in rural areas and in the oldest age groups (Figures 5-12 and 5-13). In the younger age groups of the rural population, after an initial slight increase, the rates decreased. In urban populations such an initial increase was not apparent for the younger male age groups, and for younger females the rates decreased throughout the period 1959–69.

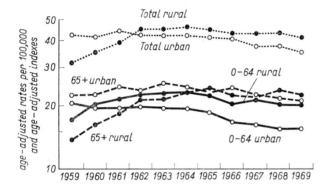

Fig. 5-12. Time trends in age-adjusted stomach cancer mortality rates and "age-adjusted indexes" up to and over 65 years of age, by urban-rural residence in the 1959–1969 period in Poland. Males.

It may be concluded from these findings that the increase of stomach cancer mortality in Poland was the result of an improvement in diagnosis whereas the risk of this cancer remained at the same level until about 1963–64 and started to decrease thereafter; the decrease began earlier for urban females.

The tendency of stomach cancer mortality to decline is probably not related to improved survival, which is very low and does not increase appreciably; only 4 percent of all stomach cancer patients survive for five years [108].

The decrease in stomach cancer mortality continued in 1970 and 1971 (Figures 4-15 and 4-16).

The trend observed in Poland differed considerably from trends in other countries [34,58,132,157]. Throughout the 1950–1965 period a distinct decrease in age-adjusted stomach cancer mortality rates was observed for both sexes in all the 24 countries presented in Figures 5-14 and 5-15, except for Japan where a decrease during the ages 40–64 has nevertheless been apparent for males since about 1955 and for females since about 1960 [160].

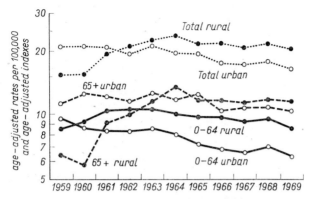

Fig. 5-13. Time trends in age-adjusted stomach cancer mortality rates and "age-adjusted indexes" up to and over 65 years of age, by urban-rural residence in the 1959–1969 period in Poland. Females.

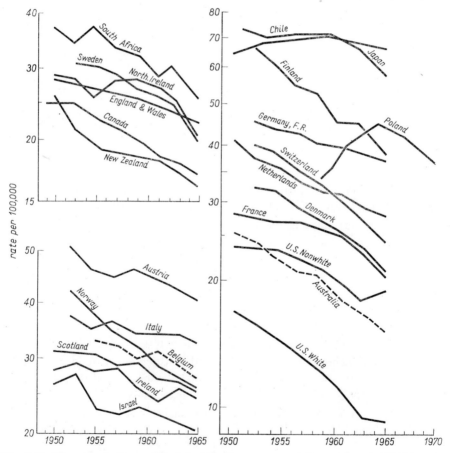

Fig. 5-14. Time trends in age-adjusted stomach cancer mortality rates, per 100,000 males, in the 1950–1965 period as reported by Segi et al.[160,161] and in the 1959–1969 period in Poland.

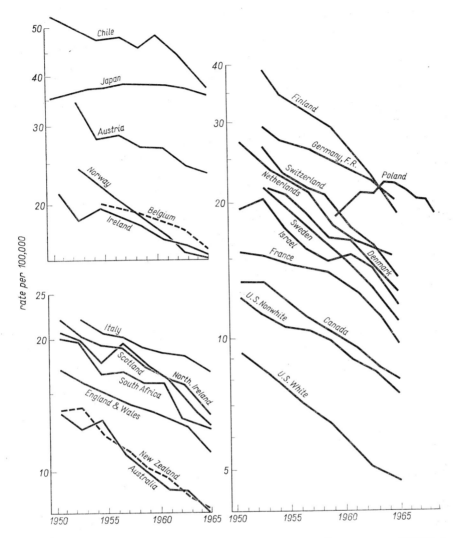

Fig. 5-15. Time trends in age-adjusted stomach cancer mortality rates, per 100,000 females, in the 1950–1965 period as reported by Segi et al.[160,161] and in the 1959–1969 period in Poland.

5.7. Polish Migrants

Except for the oldest age groups, stomach cancer mortality in Poland in 1959–61 was approximately four or five times as high as it was among native white Americans of both sexes (Figures 5-16 and 5-17). In 1950 Polish-born migrants to the United States experienced about the same mortality as prevailed in Poland in 1959–61 and had presumably prevailed in 1950 as well judging by the trends after 1959. Ten years later, however, their mortality rates decreased, becoming inter-

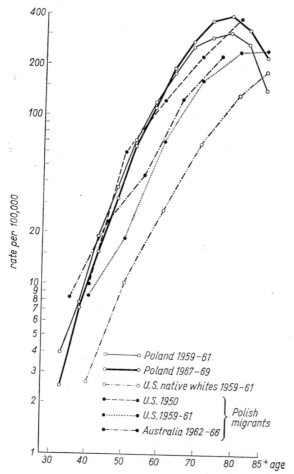

Fig. 5-16. Age-specific stomach cancer mortality rates, per 100,000 males, in Poland, in Polish migrants to the United States and to Australia, and in native white Americans.

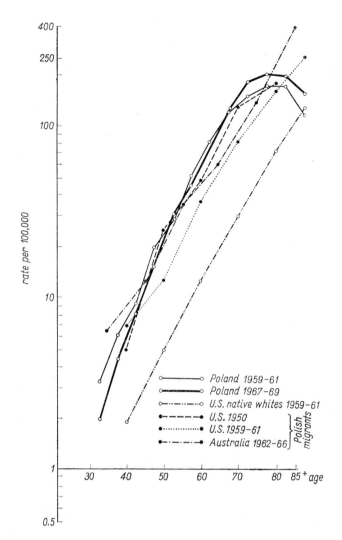

rate per 100,000

400
250

100

10

1

0.5

○———○ Poland 1959-61
●———● Poland 1967-69
○—··—··—○ U.S. native whites 1959-61
●———● U.S. 1950
●··········● U.S. 1959-61
●—·—·—● Australia 1962-66

Polish migrants

30   40   50   60   70   80   85⁺ age

Fig. 5-17. Age-specific stomach cancer mortality rates, per 100,000 females, in Poland, in Polish migrants to the United States and to Australia, and in native white Americans.

mediate between the rates in their country of origin and their country of adoption. In Australia too the 1962–66 mortality of Polish migrants was intermediate [181]; but, even though the Australian data were a few years more recent, mortality was closer to that prevailing in Poland than was the experience of the migrants to the United States.

In other migrant populations the stomach cancer mortality rates were also noted to be similar to those of their country of origin. Around 1950, mortality rates of migrants from other European countries and Japan to the United States were intermediate between the rates prevailing in their respective countries of birth and in their host country but were much closer to the rates in their countries of birth [60,65]. Ten years later stomach cancer mortality rates decreased not only in migrants from Poland, but also in Japanese [65] as well as in all foreign born inhabitants of New York City [194]. Second generation Japanese migrants to the United States, Nisei, seem to experience a further decrease of stomach cancer risk, which remains higher, however, than in native whites [65].

5.8. Discussion

5.8.1. Two Types of Stomach Cancer

Before an attempt at interpretation of the results presented above is made, an important nosologic problem will be discussed. More and more observations are corroborating the view that there are at least two types of stomach cancer, differing in histopathologic as well as epidemiologic features. Two such types were described by Laurén [107]: a diffuse and an intestinal type. It seems that whereas the first shows no significant geographic variation or time trends, the intestinal type is more prevalent in countries with high stomach cancer risk, and is becoming infrequent in low risk countries [125,126,127]. Intestinal metaplasia of the stomach epithelium, which occurs even during adolescence, with frequency and spread increasing with age, and frequently coexists with cancer of the intestinal type, is more frequent in populations with a high stomach cancer risk and seems to be a good measure of that risk. Intestinal metaplasia is considered to be a possible precancerous lesion [31,127], and it is assumed that it is connected with noninflammatory atrophy of the stomach mucosa [201]. Such atrophy can be induced experimentally by feeding low-protein diets, and also by feeding 3-methylcholanthrene [31].

Epidemiologic observations may be used to evaluate the relative importance of the genetic and environmental factors in the etiopathogenesis of stomach cancer.

5.8.2. Genetic Factors

The most important observations pointing toward a dependence of stomach cancer risk upon genetic factors come from studies of the familial aspects of this neoplasm and of the relationship between stomach cancer and blood groups [217].

Stomach cancer patients report this cancer in their families approximately twice as often as it might be expected from its occurrence in general population [217]. It is difficult to determine, however, how much these familial aggregations depend on genetic factors and how much on a common environment. Comparative studies of mono- and dizygotic twins indicate that genetic factors are rather of secondary importance in determining cancer risk [70].

Persons with blood group A have a 20 percent greater stomach cancer risk than others [22,213]; but there are indications that this association with blood group A may be limited to the diffuse type of stomach cancer [32].

Genetic factors do not account for the decreasing frequency of stomach cancer occurrence, observed in most countries. If changes of stomach cancer risk in migrant populations are also considered, genetic factors do not account for the large geographic difference in the occurrence of this cancer, too. Considering the differing epidemiologic features of both morphological types of stomach cancer, however, it is possible that the species disposition, characteristic for Man, determines the occurrence of the diffuse type of stomach cancer, whereas the intestinal type depends mainly on environmental factors.

5.8.3. Environmental Factors: Diet

Little is known yet about environmental factors predisposing to stomach cancer. The belief that dietary factors are the most important is widespread [20]; but attempts to define the specific factors in the diet of persons who develop this cancer have brought meager results [20,73,217]. One of the few positive findings is the observation of an increased risk in Poland for persons eating potatoes at least once a day [178]. This corraborates the findings of Graham et al. [56] in an area with many Polish migrants. An increased risk for persons eating much rice was found in Japan [159], and a positive correlation was noticed between cereal consumption per capita and stomach cancer mortality in 16 countries [69]. These findings may support the hypothesis that alimentary deficiences resulting from low quality diets, rich in potatoes, rice or other cereals, and poor in animal proteins, and vitamins cause a predisposition to stomach cancer [59,213,217].

It has also been postulated that stomach cancer risk may be increased by the presence in food of carcinogenic hydrocarbons created by smoke-curing or frying, of nitrosamines or their precursors, of aflatoxins or similar organic compounds, by excessive use of salt, or by distorted proportions of trace elements related to the soil or water such as a high zinc to copper ratio [7,20,43,66,85,135,152,163,192]. Present knowledge of stomach cancer epidemiology does not permit a differentiation among these hypotheses.

High stomach cancer risk in Poland is consistent with the assumption that this risk is increased by poor quality diet rich in potatoes but poor in animal proteins, fresh fruits and vegetables. The decrease in stomach cancer risk that appears to be beginning in Poland, may be due to improvement in the population's diet, an improvement noticeable since about 1950 (Appendix Table 22). It should be remembered that this amelioration was greatest for the lowest socioeconomic classes, i.e. for those with the highest stomach cancer risk. The conspicuous, characteristic for this neoplasm, negative correlation between socioeconomic class and stomach cancer [10,54,197,213], also suggests an association between stomach cancer risk and dietary deficiencies. The higher risk of this cancer in rural rather than urban population in Poland might be related to the low socioeconomic level of the rural population prevailing until after the Second World War.

None of these observations, however, exclude the hypothesis that not dietary deficiencies but food carcinogens are of primary importance in stomach cancer development. An association between eating pickled and fermented foods and stomach cancer risk was recently observed in Japan and in Japanese migrants [66]. It is possible that some microorganisms causing fermentation or accompanying it produce carcinogens [85]. An increased risk of stomach cancer in persons who like sour foods, observed in Poland [178], may perhaps be caused by increased consumption of sauerkraut, pickled cucumbers, sour milk, and the like. It is also possible that the storage of potatoes throughout winter in root cellars may favor their infection by moulds, which in turn might produce carcinogens.

5 8.4. Other Possible Environmental Factors

An association between atmospheric pollution and stomach cancer has mainly been reported in the United Kingdom where stomach cancer risk is higher in urban than in rural populations [10,20] *. The geographic pattern and decreasing occurrence of stomach cancer make it unlikely that, outside of the United Kingdom, atmospheric pollution is an important factor for this cancer. It is possible, however, that only some specific air pollutants increase the stomach cancer risk or that this effect may also depend on the coexistence of some other conditions or factors.

The association between tobacco smoking and stomach cancer is often denied. Our investigations, however, indicate that smoking increases stomach cancer risk by about 60 percent and that the increased risk pertains to cancer of the cardia and prepyloric area only [174]. Cancer of the cardia is relatively frequent in males, with an M/F ratio of about 5 : 1, which suggests an association with smoking [48]. The decreasing frequency of stomach cancer occurrence argues against such an association. It is possible, however, as Correa [31] has suggested, that this decrease is due to decreasing exposure to factors causing intestinal metaplasia of the stomach mucosa. Tobacco smoking may promote the development of cancer from the metaplastic mucosa but have no carcinogenic effect on the unchanged stomach mucosa. Such an hypothesis is supported by the observation that an association

---

* It was also reported for Łódź in Poland [19] but not corroborated by findings from other areas of Poland. The high air pollution in Katowice District was not accompanied by an increased frequency of stomach cancer occurrence.

between smoking and stomach cancer was found mainly in countries with a high frequency of this cancer — and presumably of intestinal metaplasia as well (Japan, Finland, Poland). Moreover, these countries are characterized by a high M/F ratio of stomach cancer mortality, which could also be explained by the association between smoking and stomach cancer.

5.8.5. Time of Operation and Distribution of Environmental Factors

Epidemiologic observations offer further clues to stomach cancer etiopathogenesis.

The small and slow changes of stomach cancer risk in migrant populations indicate either the primary importance of factors operating early in life or the slow change of these factors — much slower than that of factors responsible for intestinal tract cancer. The first hypothesis is supported by the parallel between the occurrence of stomach cancer and of intestinal metaplasia even at young age; this observation, reported by Correa for Colombia [31], requires confirmation by studies of other populations. In favor of the second hypothesis is the observation that, like the stomach cancer risk, the dietary habits of migrants tend to remain close to those in the country of origin. This fact has been established for Japanese migrants [62] and is probably true also for the Polish-born Americans *.

The apparent beginning of a decrease in stomach cancer mortality in Poland in recent years indicates that the prevalence of factors bearing on stomach cancer risk is decreasing. These factors seem to be distributed rather uniformly throughout the country, as may be judged from the lack of major regional differences of stomach cancer mortality in Poland.

* In 1964 in Buffalo, N.Y., I collected information on the dietary habits of Polish migrants. Most of those interviewed belonged to the second generation of migrants. From the data collected it appeared that the first, "old" generation of migrants retained dietary habits similar to those in the country of origin. The second generation, however, after eating in childhood as their parents did, soon switched to the American dietary habits when they left home.

6 | Intestinal Tract Cancer

6.1. Opening Remarks

Cancer of the small intestine and of the colon (Nos. 152 and 153, *International Classification of Diseases, ICD*, Seventh Revision, 1955) will be considered jointly because they were not separated in some of the source tabulations. They will be called cancer of the colon, because cancer of the small intestine is only a negligible part of the total.

Cancer of the rectum (No. 154, *ICD*) is usually classified separately. Distinction between colon and rectum cancer, however, is not always simple nor uniformly made in both incidence and mortality data. A substantial part of all neoplasms of the intestinal tract is located in the sigmoid colon or in the rectum, so that even a slight difference in the interpretation and application of classification rules can greatly alter the results of intestinal tract cancer classification and distort comparisons of data from various sources. Colon and rectum cancer will therefore be discussed under one heading, but their separation will be attempted.

In 1967–69 in Poland cancer of the intestinal tract was the cause of 5.5 percent of all cancer deaths in males and 6.7 percent in females. It constituted between 4 and 8 percent of all cancers reported in 1965–66 in cancer registries in the four selected areas.

The curability of intestinal tract cancer is relatively high, but varies from one geographic area to another. For example, it is higher in the United States than in Scandinavian countries [79]. In the comparison of cancer occurrence in various populations, such differences in curability can lead to discrepancies between evaluations based on mortality and morbidity statistics. Such discrepancies should be larger for intestinal tract cancer than for cancer of the stomach or lung and may be in the order of magnitude of several percentage points of the values compared.

6.2. Poland and Other Countries

Compared with mortality rates in 24 countries in 1964–65, Poland's would occupy a place close to the last for both colon and rectum cancer (Figures 6-1 and 6-2). Incidence data also indicate a low risk of colorectal cancer in Poland, with Po-

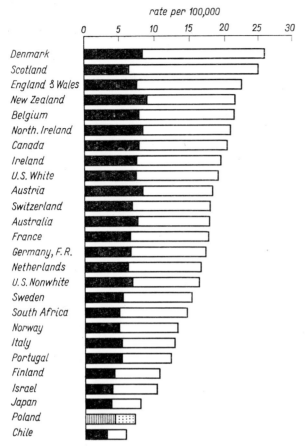

rate per 100,000

Fig. 6-1. Age-adjusted intestinal tract cancer (Nos. 152–154, *ICD*, 1955 rev.) mortality rates, per 100,000 males, in 1964–65 in 24 countries [161] and in Poland. Shaded areas represent mortality under the age of 65.

land rather low in a low-risk group consisting of Colombia, Puerto Rico, India, Japan, Hungary, Romania, and Slovenia. Only Nigeria and Rhodesia reported a significantly lower incidence [41].

In Polish 1967–69 mortality data the colon-rectum ratio, C/R, was 1.4 : 1. In the 1965–66 incidence data from the four Polish registries the lowest C/R ratio, 0.9 : 1, was observed in Katowice District; in Kraków District the C/R ratio was 1.3 : 1, and in Warszawa City, 1.5 : 1. In most countries the C/R ratio is higher than in Poland, the typical range of values being between 1.5–2.5 : 1. An exception is Japan, where the C/R ratio is only 0.7 : 1 because of the very low frequency of colon cancer whereas frequency of cancer of the rectum is not much lower there than in most other countries [65].

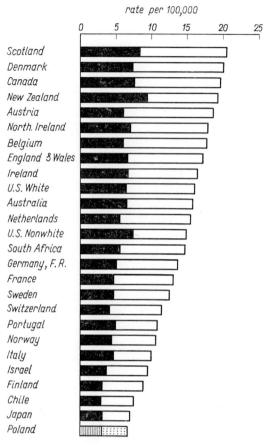

Fig. 6-2. Age-adjusted intestinal tract cancer (Nos. 152–154, *ICD*, 1955 rev.) mortality rates, per 100,000 females, in 1964–65 in 24 countries [161] and in Poland. Shaded areas represent mortality under the age of 65.

6.3. Sex

Colon cancer mortality in Poland was somewhat higher in males than in females, and the M/F ratio of about 1.1 : 1 did not change throughout the 1959–69 period. The M/F ratio was about 1.0–1.2 : 1 in most age groups, and below 1 : 1 in the oldest (Figure 6-3).

Colon cancer is one of the few non-genital cancers found more frequently in females, at least in some populations. An M/F ratio below 1 : 1 is found in just over half of the countries tabulated by Segi et al. [161]; in 22 out of 24 countries the M/F ratios ranged between 0.9–1.1 : 1. It seems that the female preponderance is diminishing, where it still exists, because of a faster increase of colon cancer risk in males. For example, among white Americans the M/F ratio increased from 0.76 : 1 in 1930–32 to 1.01 : 1 in 1964–65 [53,161].

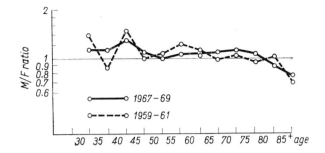

Fig. 6-3. Male/female ratios, M/F, of the age-specific colon cancer (Nos. 152–153, *ICD*, 1955 rev.) mortality rates, in 1959–61 and 1967–69 in Poland.

Rectal cancer was also more frequent in males than in females in the 1959–69 period in Poland, but the M/F ratio of 1.4 : 1, unchanged throughout that period, was higher than the ratio for colon cancer. For most age groups the M/F ratio for rectal cancer was about 1.5 : 1, but was below 1 : 1 at the age of 35–50 (Figure 6-4). Such a bimodal relation between age and M/F ratio, with the lowest values about age 35–50, is seen also in other countries, including England and Wales, Western Germany, Japan and the United States [12]. In the mortality data from 24 countries compiled by Segi et al. [161], the M/F ratio ranged between 1.0–2.2 : 1; but in 19 of those countries it ranged between 1.4–1.8 : 1.

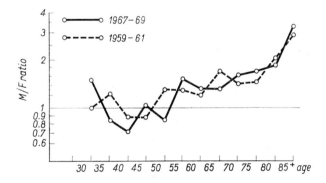

Fig. 6-4. Male/female ratios, M/F, of the age-specific rectum cancer mortality rates, in 1959–61 and 1967–69 in Poland.

6.4. Age

Mortality from intestinal tract cancer as well as its incidence usually increases with age up to the oldest age groups [37]. The rate of that increase in Poland is similar to that in other countries. Peculiar to Poland is the down-turn of the mortality-by-age curve at the age of about 70 (Figures 6-5 and 6-6), which is similar to the curve for stomach cancer and is most probably a result of the less precise certification of the causes of death in older age groups.

In Poland, as in other countries [12], the rate of mortality increase with age for colon cancer is similar for both sexes, but rectum cancer mortality increases with age faster for males than for females.

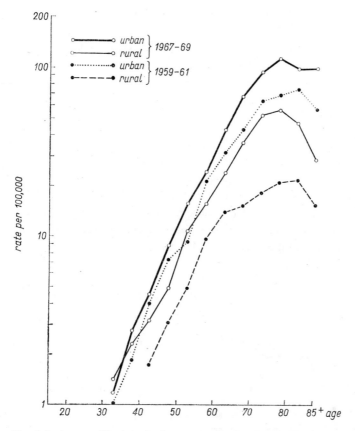

Fig. 6-5. Age-specific intestinal tract cancer (Nos. 152–154, *ICD*, 1955 rev.) mortality rates, per 100,000 males, by urban-rural residence in 1959–61 and 1967–69 in Poland.

6.5. Residence

In 1967–69, Polish age-adjusted mortality rates from intestinal·tract cancer were higher in the urban than in the rural population by 62 percent: by 76 percent for males and 46 percent for females. In the 1959–69 period the urban-rural ratio decreased in all age groups (Figures 6-7 and 6-8).

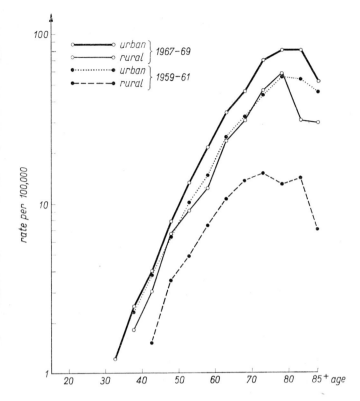

Fig. 6-6. Age-specific intestinal tract cancer (Nos. 152–154, *ICD*, 1955 rev.) mortality rates, per 100,000 females, by urban-rural residence in 1959–61 and 1967–69 in Poland.

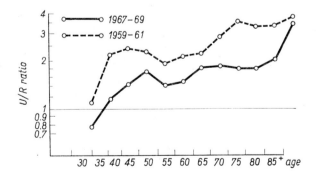

Fig. 6-7. Urban/rural ratios, U/R, of the age-specific intestinal tract cancer (Nos. 152–154, *ICD*, 1955 rev.) mortality rates, in 1959–61 and 1967–69 in Poland. Males.

6*

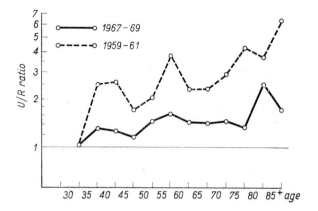

Fig. 6-8. Urban-rural ratios, U/R, of the age-specific intestinal tract cancer (Nos. 152–154, *ICD*, 1955 rev.) mortality rates, in 1959–61 and 1967–69 in Poland. Females

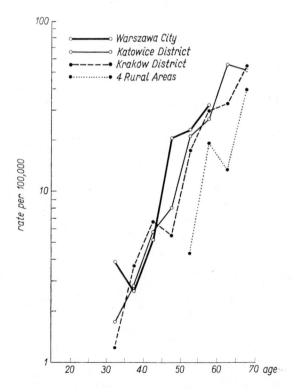

Fig. 6-9. Age-specific intestinal tract cancer (Nos. 152–154, *ICD*, 1955 rev.) incidence rates, per 100,000 males, in 1965–66 in the four regions of Poland.

The urban-rural gradient can also be observed in the incidence data, especially for colon cancer, with highest rates in Warszawa, intermediate rates in the Katowice and Kraków areas, and lowest in the rural areas. This gradient is less marked for rectal cancer, for which the Katowice area shows an incidence similar to Warszawa, but higher than in Kraków and the rural areas (Figures 6-9 and 6-10, Appendix Tables 3, 4, 5, 6).

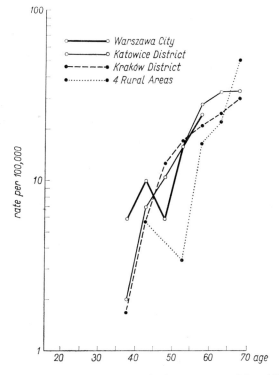

Fig. 6-10. Age-specific intestinal tract cancer (Nos. 152–154, *ICD*, 1955 rev.) incidence rates, per 100,000 females, in 1965–66 in the four regions of Poland.

Higher urban risk of colorectal cancer is also seen in other countries including Denmark, Finland, Norway, England, and the United States, where it is 25–50 percent higher than in rural areas; the urban-rural ratio was, as a rule, somewhat higher for males [118,132,218].

In 1959–61, as well as in 1967–69, the highest mortality rates for both cancers were observed in the metropolitan cities and in Katowice and Opole Districts; the lowest rates were encountered in the eastern districts (Appendix Table 18, Figures 6-11 and 6-12). Registration data are also consistent with a relatively high risk in Katowice District.

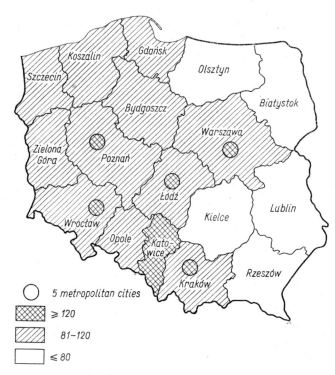

Fig. 6-11. Standardized mortality ratios, SMR, for intestinal tract cancer (Nos. 152–154, *ICD*, 1955 rev.), by district of residence in 1967–69 in Poland. Males. SMR = 100 for the total Polish population of the same sex and in the same period.

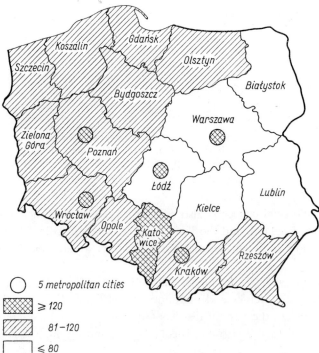

Fig. 6-12. Standardized mortality ratios, SMR, for intestinal tract cancer (Nos. 152–154, *ICD*, 1955 rev.), by district of residence in 1967–69 in Poland. Females. SMR = 100 for the total Polish population of the same sex and in the same period.

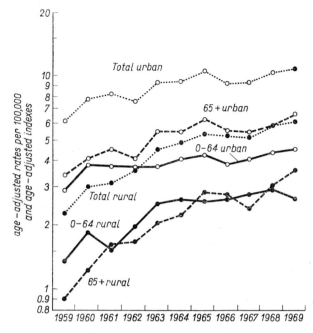

Fig. 6-13. Time trends in age-adjusted intestinal tract cancer (Nos. 152–154, *ICD,* 1955 rev.) mortality rates and "age-adjusted indexes" up to and over 65 years of age, by urban-rural residence in the 1959–1969 period in Poland. Males.

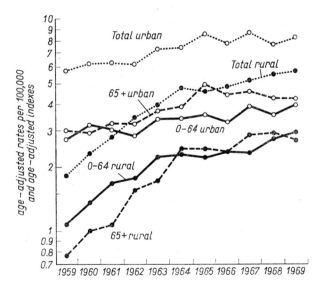

Fig. 6-14. Time trends in age-adjusted intestinal tract cancer (Nos. 152–154, *ICD,* 1955 rev.) mortality rates and "age-adjusted indexes" up to and over 65 years of age, by urban-rural residence in the 1959–1969 period in Poland. Females.

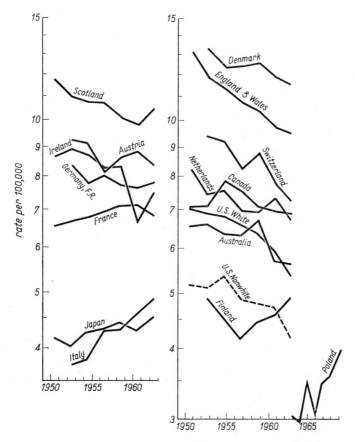

Fig. 6-15. Time trends in age-adjusted rectum cancer mortality rates, per 100,000 males, in the 1950–1965 period as reported by Segi et al.[160,161] and in the 1959–1969 period in Poland.

6.6. Time Trends

The age-adjusted mortality rates increased between 1959–69 for colon as well as for rectal cancer. The increase affected all age groups, but was more marked in the oldest, as well as in the rural population and in the first half of the period discussed (Figures 6-13 and 6-14). It seems that the increase is only partly due to the improvement of diagnosis most marked in the oldest and in the rural population, but is also partly caused by an increasing risk of intestinal tract cancer in Poland. The increase in colorectal cancer mortality was apparent also in 1970 and 1971 (Figures 4-15 and 4-16).

The increase in the intestinal tract cancer mortality, observed in Poland, is even more conspicuous if compared with data from other countries [34,53,157]. During the

1950–1965 period, rectal cancer mortality decreased in about a third of the 24 countries reported by Segi et al. [160,161] and increased distinctly in two, Japan and Italy — both with low mortality (Figures 6-15 and 6-16). Similar, but less pronounced trends in colon cancer mortality were also observed (Figures 6-17 and 6-18). Gordon et al. [58] have shown that mortality rates of white Americans initially increased in the 1930–1955 period — for rectal cancer until 1945 and for colon cancer until 1940 — but declined thereafter.

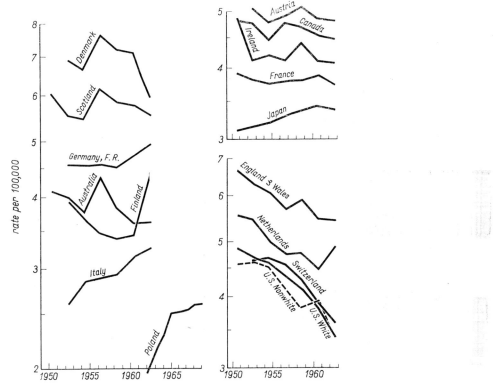

Fig. 6-16. Time trends in age-adjusted rectum cancer mortality rates, per 100,000 females, in the 1950–1965 period as reported by Segi et al. [160,161] and in the 1959–1969 period in Poland.

Comparing trends in incidence, mortality and survival rates in the United States in the 1935–1965 period, Cutler [34] has shown that the decrease of rectal cancer mortality was due at first to improved survival, but after 1955 to decreasing incidence of the disease. On the other hand, the increasing incidence of colon cancer was not accompanied by a rising mortality rate because it was offset by improved survival resulting both from more frequent performance of surgical treatment and from improvement of treatment results.

In Norway colon cancer incidence increased by 41 percent in males and 30 percent in females between 1955 and 1967, whereas rectum cancer incidence increased by 16 and 19 percent, respectively. The increase was fairly uniform for all ages [195].

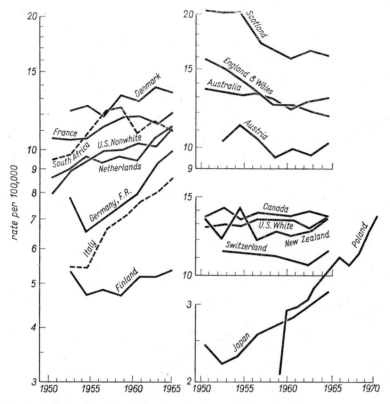

Fig. 6-17. Time trends in age-adjusted colon cancer (Nos. 152–153, *ICD*, 1955 rev.) mortality rates, per 100,000 males, in the 1950–1965 period as reported by Segi et al. [160,161] and in the 1959–1969 period in Poland.

6.7. Polish Migrants

Polish-born Americans experienced colon and rectal cancer mortality rates higher than those of native white Americans (Figures 6-19 and 6-20), but similar to the rates in the northeast and north central states, where the rates are above the United States average [60] and where most Polish migrants reside. This finding corroborates an earlier conclusion based on data for 1950 only — that mortality for these cancers among Polish-born migrants is much higher than in Poland and similar to that of United States natives [180]. It is worth remarking that Polish migrants to the United States were drawn mainly from the farming, rural areas, those areas where the risk of these cancers was probably even below the low Polish average.

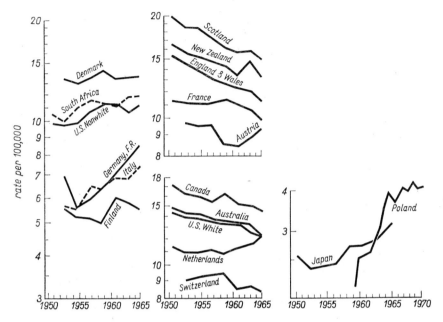

Fig. 6-18. Time trends in age-adjusted colon cancer (Nos. 152–153, *ICD*, 1955 rev.) mortality rates, per 100,000 females, in the 1950–1965 period as reported by Segi et al. [160,161] and in the 1959–1969 period in Poland.

The upward displacement of the colorectal cancer risk for those migrants was thus probably even larger than seems from the rates presented.

A similar increase of the intestinal tract cancer mortality, connected with migration from a low risk to a high risk area for this cancer, was observed in the United States in migrants from Norway and Japan [65], as well as from rural to urban areas, whereas mortality decreased in migrants from urban to rural areas [64]. The colorectal cancer risk of migrants appears to be related more to the risk prevailing in their last residence area than to the risk in their country of birth.

Among Polish migrants to Australia a similar increase of colon and rectal cancer mortality to the high level prevailing in their country of adoption was observed. That increase was admittedly small among males; but this deviation may be the result of chance variation, the male rates being based on only 20 deaths.

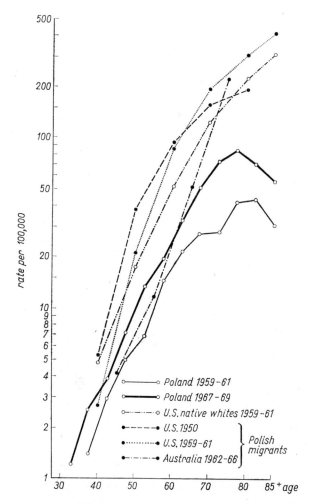

Fig. 6-19. Age-specific intestinal tract cancer (Nos. 152–154, *ICD*, 1955 rev.) mortality rates, per 100,000 males, in Poland, in Polish migrants to the United States and to Australia, and in native white Americans.

6.8. Discussion

6.8.1. Localization

Some observations indicate that cancers of different parts of the colon and rectum may have distinct epidemiologic features. It appears, for example, that the frequency of occurrence of cancer of the distal part of the rectum is similar in Japan and in Japanese migrants in Hawaii, whereas the frequency of cancer of the proximal part of the rectum and of the distal part of the colon is much higher in those

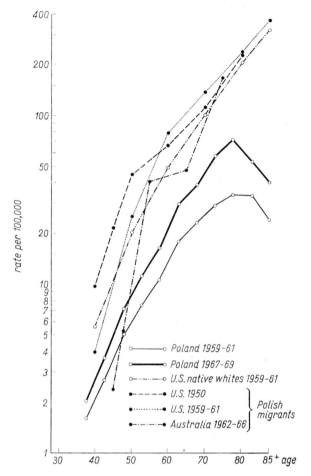

Fig. 6-20. Age-specific intestinal tract cancer (Nos. 152–154, *ICD*, 1955 rev.) mortality rates, per 100,000 females, in Poland, in Polish migrants to the United States and to Australia, and in native white Americans.

migrants than in their country of birth [187,188]. The increase of intestinal tract cancer risk in Japanese migrants to the United States may thus be explained mainly by the increase of rectosigmoid junction cancer risk. This would corroborate the hypothesis that when a new etiologic factor is introduced into a low-risk population, the transition from an "endemic" to an "epidemic" phase is first expressed as a rise in sigmoid cancers [63].

Studies of the epidemiologic characteristics of cancers of different parts of the intestinal tract unfortunately are hindered by the paucity and insufficient precision of data on the occurrence of tumors in various segments of the colon and rectum.

A little more is known about the epidemiologic differences between colon and rectum cancer. The differences in the sex ratios were stressed in section 6.3. More difficult is the interpretation of geographic differences in the colon-rectum ratio, C/R, because classification of the frequent "border" cases may vary between the geographic areas compared *. However, studies of migrant populations indicate that at least some of the geographic differences in the C/R ratio are real, and not due to varying classification practices.

The low C/R ratio in Poland, about 1.4 : 1, is corroborated by a slightly higher C/R ratio of 1.6 : 1, noticed in Polish migrants in the United States in 1950; this ratio increased over the next 10 years to 2.7 : 1, the level prevailing among native Americans. Also in Japanese migrants to the United States the C/R ratio of only 2.0 : 1, lower than in native Americans, corroborates the low C/R ratio observed in Japan [65].

A better knowledge of tumor localization would be useful not only in identifying the possible epidemiologic differences between cancers of different segments of the intestinal tract, but also in clarifying the relation between polyps and cancer of the intestinal tract [3,24,63]. Results of a comparative study, conducted in Colombia and United States, indicate that intestinal polyps are more frequent in the left than in the right colon in countries in which intestinal tract cancer risk is high, whereas in low-risk countries such polyps appear more frequently in the right colon [33,63].

Among precancerous conditions are ulcerative colitis and familial polyposis, but only a small proportion of intestinal tract cancers is related to these conditions [36,218].

Knowledge about factors bearing on intestinal tract cancer risk is still very incomplete.

6.8.2. Genetic Factors

These seem to be of some importance here, as indicated by the increased risk in persons with familial polyposis. Intestinal tract cancer is also more frequent than expected, assuming independence from familial factors, in families of patients with this cancer. How far this depends on genetic factors or on a common environment is hard to tell. No association with blood groups has been demonstrated [218].

Large geographic variation in the frequency of intestinal tract cancer occurrence, and the substantial changes in risk observed in migrant populations, indicate that environmental factors are more important than genetic ones for the etiopathogenesis of this cancer.

6.8.3. Environmental Factors

It is frequently assumed that dietary factors may operate either directly, acting as carcinogens on the intestinal mucosa, or indirectly, influencing intestinal bacteria or peristalsis. Possible dietary carcinogens might be present in food in an active

* Two recent studies indicate that the actual differences in assignement of the recto-sigmoid cancer cases to colon or to rectum explain only a minor part of the observed variation in C/R ratio (De Jong et al., *Int. J. Cancer* 10, 463, 1972; Haenszel and Correa [63]).

form or, more likely, might be activated in the intestines by the bacteria. For instance, it was shown experimentally that in rats fed with cycasin intestinal cancer develops only in the presence of intestinal bacteria [106]. It also seems that intestinal bacteria may transform biliary salts into carcinogens [8].

Intestinal bacteria are dependent on diet, especially on relative proportions of fats and carbohydrates [215,218]. Hence, it can be expected that the possible activation of food carcinogens by intestinal bacteria may also be diet dependent.

The low frequency of intestinal tract cancer occurrence in populations with bulky diets [21,73] is consistent with the hypothesis that the risk of this cancer is decreased by factors which increase peristalsis and thus decrease the contact of intestinal mucosa with carcinogens present in intestinal contents. Such an hypothesis would explain the negative correlation of these neoplasms with tobacco smoking, since nicotine increases peristalsis [174].

Evaluation of the relative importance of the possible ways in which diet may influence the development of intestinal tract cancer is made difficult by their interrelations. For example a diet rich in fats is usually not bulky and thus does not promote peristalsis; bacteria associated with such a diet differ also from the bacteria associated with a high carbohydrate diet; moreover, fats increase bile excretion, and biliary salts may possibly be transformed into carcinogens by intestinal bacteria.

The low, but increasing risk of intestinal tract cancer in Poland may be a result of the high, but decreasing consumption of potatoes, which are rich in cellulose, provide bulky food and promote peristalsis; it may also be related to the low, but increasing consumption of fats or sugar because of their effect on intestinal bacteria or on the supply of materials from which carcinogen is made.

Bulky, low-fat diets are usually qualitatively poor and low in animal proteins and vitamins. This might explain the negative correlation between cancers of the intestinal tract and of the stomach.

There is a positive correlation between colon cancer and coronary heart disease [65,218]. The increased risk of both diseases may depend on dietary habits including an excessive intake of fats, especially animal fats, combined with obesity and lack of physical activity which create a predisposition to constipation.

Recently a negative correlation between colon cancer and cerebro-vascular accidents, CVA, was noticed. The best examples of the phenomenon are Japan, where there are exceptionally high CVA and low colon cancer mortality; and Japanese migrants to the United States among whom CVA mortality became low, whereas colon cancer mortality came to be high [65]. Here too change of environment, and especially of dietary habits, may be suspected as the common factor.

A positive correlation also exists between intestinal tract cancer and cancer of the breast, corpus uteri, and ovary [49,154,214].

The rapid change in risk among Polish migrants shows that, for intestinal tract cancer development, the environment in the last place of residence is much more important than the environment in childhood or adolescence. Also the results of a study of the effects of internal migration in the United States indicate that the intestinal tract cancer risk of migrants is similar to the risk experienced by the native-born residents of the host area rather than to the risk prevailing in the place of the migrants' birth [64]. Displacement of risk for intestinal tract cancer in migrants thus follows a different pattern from that observed for stomach cancer. Whereas stomach cancer mortality among Polish-born Americans first began to decline after 1950 but in 1959–61 was still closer to the level prevailing in their country of birth, their intestinal tract cancer mortality had already reached the level of their host country by 1950. Several hypotheses might account for this difference in behavior of the risks of cancers of the adjacent parts of the alimentary canal:

a) factors influencing cancer risks for the stomach persist and carry over unchanged for a long time in the new environment, but do not do so for intestinal tract cancer;

b) change in or withdrawal of factors influencing cancer risk coincide with change of residence; this change comes too late to halt initiated stomach cancer but early enough to induce or to withdraw inhibition of induction of intestinal tract cancer;

c) "migrant" effects for these cancers are expressed in one direction only, through moves from low-risk to high-risk areas.

The last hypothesis is the least likely because a decrease of intestinal tract cancer risk was also observed in United States migrants from urban to rural areas [64]; that single observation, however, requires confirmation.

Intestinal tract cancer is currently much less of a problem in Poland than stomach cancer. The trends observed in Poland, however, and in other countries, strongly suggest that in Poland too, intestinal tract cancer will soon become one of the most frequent cancers. This should be kept in mind in planning the organization of cancer diagnosis and treatment, as well as in the search for measures for cancer prevention.

7 | Lung Cancer

7.1. Opening Remarks

In 1967–69, lung cancer accounted for 22.3 percent of all cancer deaths among all Polish males, ranking second after stomach cancer, and for urban males it ranked first among causes of cancer death. Results of the registration of new cancer cases in the selected regions of Poland in 1965–66 are similar: lung cancer was the most frequent cancer in Warszawa City in males, and second most frequent in the other three regions (Appendix Tables 3, 4, 5, 6).

In 1971 lung cancer became the most frequent cause of cancer death in Polish males, outranking stomach cancer for the first time (Figure 4-15).

For females, lung cancer was the cause of 4.7 percent of cancer deaths in 1967–69.

Mortality and morbidity statistics render similar estimates of lung cancer occurrence because of the low curability of this cancer and the short survival period after its diagnosis.

7.2. Poland and Other Countries

Compared with lung cancer mortality in 24 countries in 1964–65, Poland would occupy the 19th place for males and 18th for females (Figures 7-1 and 7-2). Cancer registration data indicate that the lung cancer incidence in comparison with other countries in Polish males is slightly above average, and in females a little below average [41].

7.3. Sex

Lung cancer mortality rates in 1959–61 in Poland were five times higher for males than for females, and in 1967–69 seven times higher. The sex ratio, M/F, rose in each age-group; in both periods it was highest between 55–75 (Figure 7-3).

In 1964–65 the M/F ratios of lung cancer mortality rates in 24 countries ranged from 3 : 1 in Japan, Chile and Israel to 16 : 1 in Finland; for most countries the

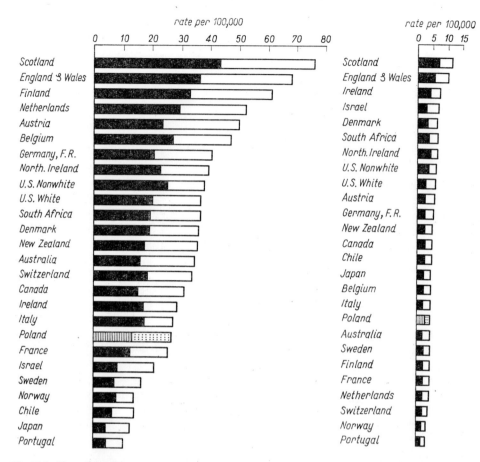

Fig. 7-1. Age-adjusted lung cancer mortality rates, per 100,000 males, in 1964–65 in 24 countries [161] and in Poland.

Fig. 7-2. Age-adjusted lung cancer mortality rates, per 100,000 females, in 1964–65 in 24 countries [161] and in Poland.

Remark to Fig. 7-1 and 7-2. Shaded areas represent mortality under the age of 65.

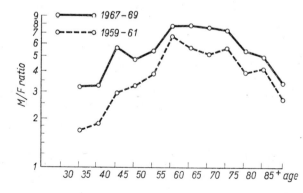

Fig. 7–3. Male/female ratios of the age-specific lung cancer mortality rates, in 1959–61 and 1967–69 in Poland.

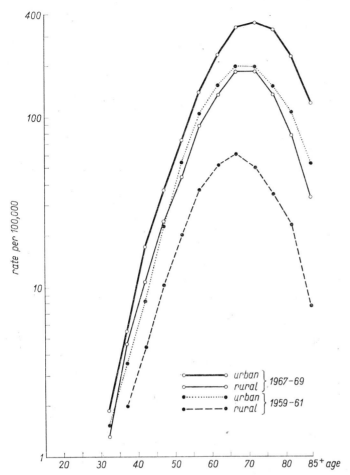

Fig. 7-4. Age-specific lung cancer mortality rates, per 100,000 males, by urban-rural residence in 1959–61 and 1967–69 in Poland.

range was about 6–9 : 1 [161]. In the first two or three decades of this century the M/F ratio was about 1.5–2 : 1, but it has risen in more recent years [165]. However, since 1960 in the United States a reversal of this trend has been observed, the result of a growing rate of lung cancer mortality in females; the M/F ratio decreased from 6.8 : 1 in 1960 to 6.1 : 1 in 1965 [196]. A similar decrease of the M/F ratio was observed in Warszawa City by Koszarowski [93].

The M/F ratio varies for different histologic types of lung cancer. For example, among 281 lung cancer patients, whose smoking habits were analyzed in 1954–58 [167], the M/F ratio was found to be 1.8 : 1 for adenocarcinoma and 24.0 : 1 for the other and unspecified histological types (only 1 out of 138 squamous cell carcinomas was encountered in a female). These findings are consistent with reports from other countries [165,196].

7*

7.4. Age

Deflection of the incidence- and mortality-by-age curve at about the age of 65 is characteristic for lung cancer in males in Poland as well as in other countries (Figures 7-4 and 7-16). Analyses of mortality statistics from a long time period, 1914–1961 in the United States [165], demonstrated this deflection to be the result of a summation of mortality of successive cohorts (persons born in the same period, say in the same five-year period). For each of these cohorts the lung cancer mortality

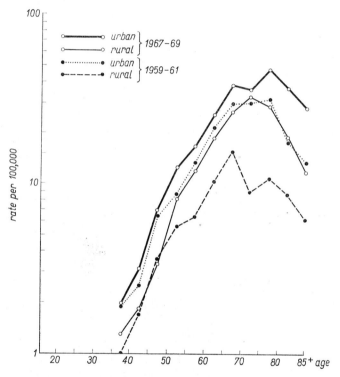

Fig. 7-5. Age-specific lung cancer mortality rates, per 100,000 females, by urban-rural residence in 1959–61 and 1967–69 in Poland.

rates increase with advancing age up to the oldest age groups, but the speed of that increase varies: the younger the cohort, the greater the speed and the steeper the slope of the mortality-by-age curve. This suggests an increasing exposure of younger cohorts to carcinogenic factors.

In females the increase of lung cancer mortality rates in younger cohorts is much smaller, hence there is usually no deflection of the mortality-by-age curve; e.g. in native white Americans (Fig. 7-17).

The slope of the mortality-by-age curve for Polish males up to the age of 60 is similar to that of other populations compared, whereas for Polish females it is steeper (Figures 7-16 and 7-17).

7.5. Residence

In Poland, as in other countries [67,118], lung cancer occurs more frequently in urban than in rural populations, and this disparity between urban and rural mortality is more evident among males than among females. The disparity decreased between 1959–61 and 1967–69. The urban-rural ratio, U/R, now equals 1.74 : 1 for males and 1.45 : 1 for females (Figures 7-6 and 7-7).

Lung cancer mortality rates above average for the country were observed for males in metropolitan cities, in western districts, and also in Katowice, Opole,

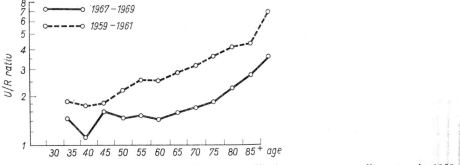

Fig. 7-6. Urban-rural ratios, U/R, of the age-specific lung cancer mortality rates, in 1959–61 and 1967–69 in Poland. Males.

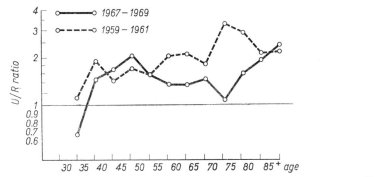

Fig. 7-7. Urban-rural ratios, U/R, of the age-specific lung cancer mortality rates, in 1959–61 and 1967–69 in Poland. Females.

Gdańsk and Bydgoszcz Districts in both 1961 [172] and 1967 (Appendix Table 18, Figure 7-8). For females, because of the small number of lung cancer deaths, when subdivided by districts, it is possible only to conclude that mortality rates were higher in metropolitan cities, whereas in Katowice District they were rather below average (Figure 7-9).

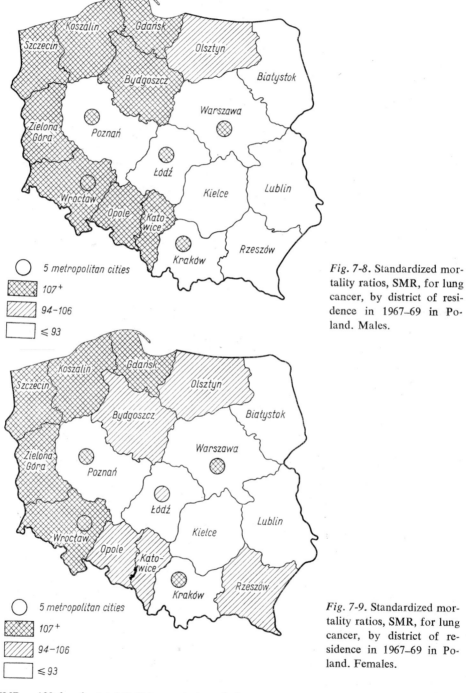

Fig. 7-8. Standardized mortality ratios, SMR, for lung cancer, by district of residence in 1967–69 in Poland. Males.

Fig. 7-9. Standardized mortality ratios, SMR, for lung cancer, by district of residence in 1967–69 in Poland. Females.

SMR = 100 for the total Polish population of the same sex and in the same period.

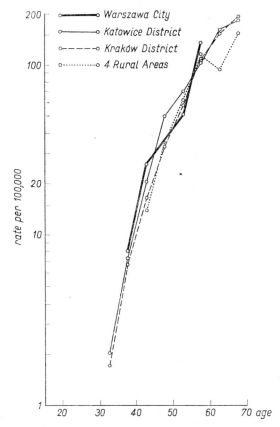

Fig. 7-10. Age-specific lung cancer incidence rates, per 100,000 males, in 1965–66 in the four regions of Poland.

The incidence of lung cancer was similar in all the four registration areas for males aged below 60, whereas for females it was highest in Warszawa City, and lowest in Katowice District (Figures 7-10 and 7-11).

7.6. Time Trends

The rapid increase in lung cancer mortality rates in males and a much slower increase in females is observed in all countries (Figures 7-14 and 7-15). Poland is no exception in this respect. Among males this increase involved all age groups, both urban and rural, but was more rapid for the rural population and for older age groups. It seems that much of that mortality increase was due to a true rise in lung cancer risk. Among females lung cancer mortality increased for the rural, and for

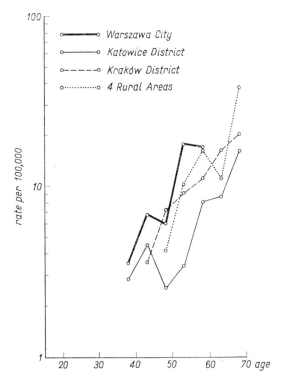

Fig. 7-11. Age-specific lung cancer incidence rates, per 100,000 females, in 1965–66 in the four regions of Poland.

the urban population aged 65 and over. Since about 1965 an increase in mortality has also been apparent for younger urban females, indicating an increase in lung cancer risk (Figures 7-12 and 7-13).

7.7. Polish Migrants

In 1950 the highest lung cancer mortality rates among males in the United States were observed among Polish-born Americans [60]. An instance of this is the observation that for patients of the Roswell Park Memorial Institute in Buffalo, N.Y., the lung cancer risk among Polish migrants was higher than that among any other ethnic group during the 1945–1956 period [55]. Although 1950 lung cancer mortality rates among males who migrated to the United States from England and Wales, Norway, Sweden, Germany and Italy were intermediate between the rates reported for their country of origin and for natives of their country of adoption [60], these

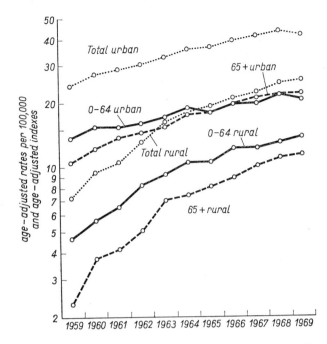

Fig. 7-12. Time trends in age-adjusted lung cancer mortality rates and "age-adjusted indexes" up to and over 65 years of age, by urban-rural residence in the 1959–1969 period in Poland. Males.

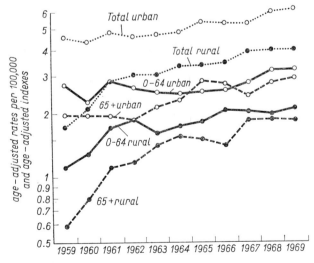

Fig. 7-13. Time trends in age-adjusted lung cancer mortality rates and "age-adjusted indexes" up to and over 65 years of age, by urban-rural residence in the 1959–1969 period in Poland. Females.

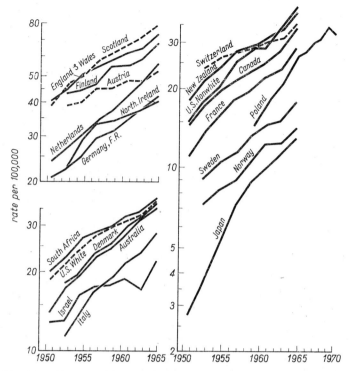

Fig. 7-14. Time trends in age-adjusted lung cancer mortality rates, per 100,000 males, in the 1950–1965 period as reported by Segi et al. [160,161] and in the 1959–1969 period in Poland.

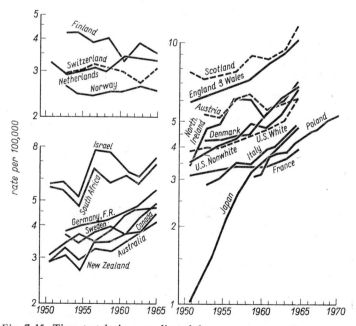

Fig. 7-15. Time trends in age-adjusted lung cancer mortality rates, per 100,000 females, in the 1950–1965 period as reported by Segi et al. [160,161] and in the 1959–1969 period in Poland.

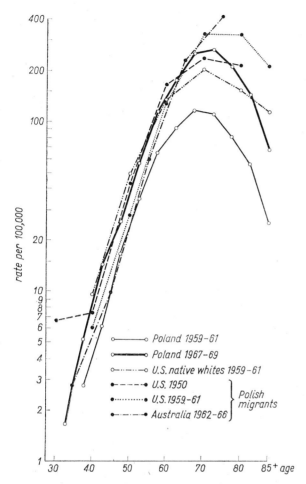

Fig. 7-16. Age-specific lung cancer mortality rates, per 100,000 males, in Poland, in Polish migrants to the United States and to Australia, and in native white Americans.

rates among Polish-born Americans were distinctly higher in all age-groups (especially 55 and over) than in either Poland or among native Americans [180]. Ten years later lung cancer mortality rates increased only for the age groups over 65 but, unexpectedly, decreased for the younger ones (Figure 7-16). Among native Americans the increase in lung cancer mortality rates was also most conspicuous in older age groups, but in the younger groups the rates did not decrease but increased. As a result, 1959–61 lung cancer mortality rates among Polish-born Americans were higher only than those for native white Americans over the age of 65, but lower for those below that age.

Lung cancer mortality rates among Polish migrants to Australia in 1962–66 were similar to the rates reported for similar years both in their countries of birth and of adoption [181].

For females who migrated from Poland to the United States, lung cancer mortality rates have increased in all age groups, except one. Both in 1950 and in 1959–61 these rates were higher than they were for native Americans by about 50 percent

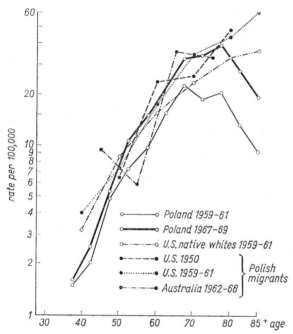

Fig. 7-17. Age-specific lung cancer mortality rates, per 100,000 females, in Poland, in Polish migrants to the United States, and to Australia, and in native white Americans.

(Appendix Table 17, Figure 7-17). Allowance for the fact that most of these migrants lived in metropolitan areas, where lung cancer mortality rates were above the country's average, reduces the excess of the rate among Polish migrants to 15 percent.

The small number of lung cancer deaths reported among Polish female migrants to Australia permits no definite conclusions concerning their cancer risk.

7.8. Discussion

7.8.1. Genetic Factors

These account neither for geographic variation nor for time trends in lung cancer occurrence which point out the importance of environmental factors in etiopathogenesis of this cancer.

7.8.2. Tobacco Smoking

The currently most important factor determining lung cancer occurrence is believed to be cigarette smoking.

A case-control study conducted 1954–58 showed that in Poland the risk of lung cancer is about 10 times higher among smokers than among nonsmokers; more than 80 percent of all cases of this cancer were estimated to be associated with smoking [167,168]. These findings closely correspond to data from other countries [165,196] and contradict the suggestion proffered by Beffinger [15,45] that tobacco processing methods in use in Poland, different from processing methods employed in western countries, decrease the carcinogenic effects of tobacco smoking.

Cigar and pipe smokers experience less lung cancer risk than cigarette smokers, probably because they usually inhale far less smoke. A relatively high incidence of pipe and cigar smoking among older males in the Katowice and Poznań areas lowers the percentage of cigarette smokers, and is probably the reason of the relatively low lung cancer mortality in these areas [172].

The increase in lung cancer mortality rates observed in Poland can be accounted for most probably by the increase in cigarette consumption and, to a lesser extent, by the improved diagnosis of this cancer, especially in rural areas and older age groups (Table 7-1).

Table 7-1

Annual per capita consumption of cigarettes in Poland — 1933–1971

Year	1933–37	1946	1947	1948	1949	1950	1951	1952	1953	1954	1955	1956
No. cigarettes[1]	672[2]	—	—	—	893	1,063	1,120	1,169	1,204	1,278	1,378	1,471

1957	1958	1959	1960	1961	1962	1963	1964	1965	1966	1967	1968	1969	1970	1971
1,511	1,552	1,566	1,539	1,649	1,683	1,677	1,661	1,700	1,790	1,844	1,967	2,074	2,082	2,217

[1] one cigarette is approximately equivalent to one gram of tobacco; after the Second World War cigarettes accounted for about 99 percent of all tobacco consumption.

[2] all tobacco products converted to the equivalent in cigarettes.

Lung cancer risk in a population seems to correspond to cigarette consumption by that population 20–30 years earlier. The three-fold increase in cigarette consumption over the past three decades in Poland foretells a further rapid increase in lung cancer mortality. This increase could be promptly impeded by a decrease in cigarette consumption: it has already been demonstrated that cessation of smoking is followed in a few years by a substantial decrease in lung cancer risk [40].

7.8.3. Occupational Exposure and General Air Pollution

Occupational exposure to uranium ores, chromium, nickel or arsen compounds, asbestos, or nitrogen mustard increases lung cancer risk, apparently more in smokers than in nonsmokers; the joint effect of both factors, occupational exposure and cigarette smoking, is not a sum but rather a product of their separate effects [112,162].

The effects of occupational exposure, like those of smoking, are more closely associated with squamous cell, oat cell and undifferentiated carcinoma than with adenocarcinoma of the lung [40,104].

Lung cancer risk is greater in urban than in rural populations. That difference slightly diminishes, but does not disappear, after an adjustment is made for differences in smoking habits. The increased risk to lung cancer in urban residents is usually considered to be the result of air pollution. It may also depend on occupational factors, as is also suggested by the higher urban-rural ratio in males than in females. It is possible, however, that the higher male U/R ratio also depends on differences in smoking habits and that the high proportion of female nonsmokers depresses the urban-rural ratio in females [67,68].

Just et al. [88] reported that in 1965–66 the aromatic hydrocarbon content in the dust in the air of 10 cities in Poland was higher than that of other European and non-European cities; it was lowest in Warszawa City and highest in Zabrze, one of the industrial cities in Katowice District. These authors point to the fact that "... aromatic hydrocarbons discovered in the air are not in themselves direct causes of respiratory cancer risks to the urban population. They are indicators of these risks".

Available data on lung cancer occurrence in Poland, especially the relatively low incidence and mortality rates reported for Katowice District, are consistent with the view that cigarette smoking is the main factor determining the lung cancer risk in Poland, and that general air pollution or occupational exposure play only a secondary role. It is nevertheless possible that, aside from the hazards of smoking, high risks may exist or soon appear in the form of occupational hazards to some small groups.

7.8.4. Migration Effect

The unexpected discovery of an increased lung cancer risk in both male and female migrants from farms * to urban areas of the United States [67,68] is indirectly supported by observation of the increased risk to the, mainly rural, Polish [180] and Japanese [63] migrants to the United States. As an explanation, two hypotheses have been advanced. One proposes a lack of adaptation in persons born on farms. "... an abrupt imposition of additional particulate matter ... from the urban atmosphere with no intervening period of gradual adaptation to an increasing load. This, when added to cigarette smoke, might overload and inhibit the action of the respiratory cilia in particle transport, and would thus permit longer contact of the particles, and any carcinogens adhering to their surfaces, with the epithelial cells" [67].

This hypothesis may be difficult to reconcile with the indications of increased risk also observed among nonsmoking migrants from farms to urban areas [67].

The other hypothesis postulates a better adaptation in the urban population rather than a lack of adaptation in the rural; exposure at birth, or even *in utero*, to small carcinogen doses might create some resistance, perhaps by preconditioning enzyme metabolism [68].

Differentiation between the implications of these two hypotheses would require knowledge of age at migration as well as at starting to smoke. The first hypothesis suggests the greatest risk for those who simultaneously migrate and start to smoke, or substantially increase smoking intensity, or switch from pipe or cigars to cigarettes; a gradual increase in smoking intensity would be followed by a lower lung cancer risk than the risk experienced by those who smoked heavily from the start. The second hypothesis would not require these conditions, but would be supported by the finding of a gradient with the lowest risk for those who migrated very early in childhood when there might still be some possibility of adaptation. Poland appears to be an adventagous place for studies designed to elucidate the migration effect on lung cancer risk. Subjects for such studies might be found not only (as elsewhere) among the numbers of young adults, especially those between 18 and 29, who frequently migrate from rural to urban areas in search of education or better jobs [78], but also (what would be of particular interest for such studies) among the large groups of Poles who were transferred during and immediately after the Second World War in a forced migration that involved all age groups including children.

Another intriguing phenomenon connected with migration is the decrease in lung cancer mortality, observed between 1950 and 1959–61 in Polish-born American males in all age groups up to 55–64. Available information is insufficient to explain this phenomenon. For example, the smoking habits of these migrants are

---

* That effect, observed in migrants to urban areas, was limited to persons born on farms, and was absent from those of nonfarm rural origin in the United States.

unknown to the author. There are indications, however, that migrants in these age groups differ from other migrants in their habits, backgrounds and other factors.

The "old" migration came predominantly from the rural, farming areas of Poland, and consisted of poor, ill-educated, often landless people; probably only few migrated as children or adolescents, and migration from Poland to the United States was virtually stopped around 1924. On the other hand, a substantial proportion of the younger age groups members probably came from the "new" migration *. These people left Poland during the time of the Second World War and arrived in the United States in the forties and fifties; thus they were only partly included in the 1950 mortality data. In contrast to the "old", the "new" migration, caused by the 1939–45 war, came mainly from just the opposite part of the society: well educated, higher socioeconomic classes, mostly from large cities.

The decrease in lung cancer mortality rates observed in the younger age groups of Polish-born Americans thus could be a result of the increased proportion of individuals from the "new" migration in these age groups, either because their cigarette consumption may be lower or because their predominantly urban background has minimized the migration effect. To differentiate between these possibilities, data on both smoking habits of Polish migrants and on their residence in their country of birth would be necessary, as well as data on their age at migration.

* Persons who were under 65 around 1960 were born after 1895; if they left Poland at the age of over 18, it means they migrated after the 1914–1918 World War. Few of those born after 1905 could have migrated between 1924 and the Second World War.

8 | Breast Cancer

8.1. Opening Remarks

During the 1967–69 period in Poland, breast cancer was certified as the cause in 10.9 percent of all cancer deaths among females, ranking third after stomach and uterus cancer. In incidence breast cancer ranked second, after cervix uteri cancer, in three out of the four selected regions of Poland, but third in the rural areas.

In males mortality as well as incidence was about one fiftieth as great as that in females, corresponding to observations made in other countries [158]. Information about breast cancer occurrence in males is based on small numbers and does not permit a detailed analysis; further discussion will be limited to breast cancer in females.

In spite of the relatively high curability of breast cancer, both morbidity and mortality statistics give similar estimates of regional differences in its occurrence [47]. A comparison of survival statistics in five countries showed only minor differences [79]. The suggestion that breast cancer prognosis is somewhat better in countries with a low frequency of occurrence [216] requires confirmation.

8.2. Poland and Other Countries

Breast cancer risk in Poland is among the lowest. Poland is third from the last in mortality, ahead of only Chile and Japan when compared with the 24 countries (Figure 8-1). A comparison of cancer incidence data also places the four Polish registers toward the bottom along with Slovenia, Hungary, Africa, Bombay in India, Cali in Colombia, and Puerto Rico [41].

8.3. Age

As with other cancers, breast cancer risk increases with age, but a characteristic feature of breast cancer is a slowing down in the rate of that increase at about the age of 45–50. Two linear components or segments are therefore discernable in the risk-by-age diagram. The first segment, up to about age 45, is the steeper one. Its slope is similar for high- and low-risk countries [82,204]. For Poland in 1967–69, compared with 1959–61, this component moved to the left, showing higher risk values for each age, but did not change slope; there is now not much difference between urban and rural areas (Figure 8-2). The second segment, on the other

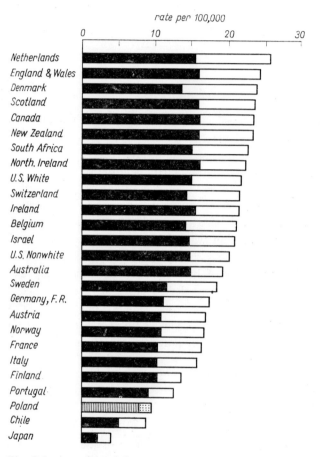

Fig. 8-1. Age-adjusted breast cancer mortality rates, per 100,000 females, in 1964–65 in 24 countries [161] and in Poland. Shaded areas represent mortality under the age of 65.

hand, which corresponds to the older age groups (postmenopausal and perhaps menopausal) has a steeper slope for countries with a high risk of this cancer than for low risk countries [82,204]. For Poland this segment is less steep than the first segment and less steep for rural than for urban populations; its slope increased more for rural than for urban females between 1959–61 and 1967–69.

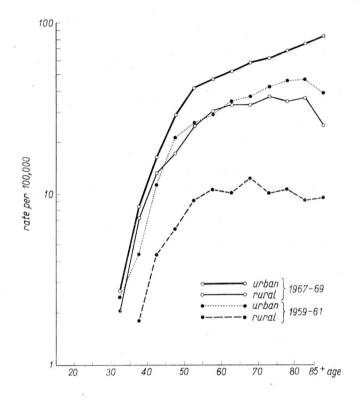

Fig. 8-2. Age-specific breast cancer mortality rates, per 100,000 females, by urban-rural residence in 1959–61 and 1967–69 in Poland.

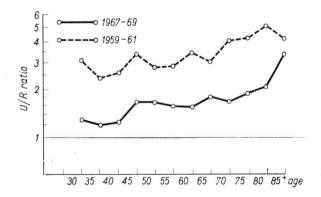

Fig. 8-3. Urban-rural ratios, U/R, of the female age-specific breast cancer mortality rates in 1959–61 and 1967–69 in Poland.

8*

8.4. Residence

Although initially large, the urban preponderance has decreased markedly in all age groups (Figure 8-3). The urban-rural mortality ratio, U/R, was 1.65 : 1 in 1967–69, although it was 3.21 : 1 in 1959–61, and 4.0 : 1 in 1952 [176].

In 1965–66 breast cancer incidence in females aged 40 and over was higher in Warszawa City than in the other three registration areas (Figure 8-4, Appendix Tables 3, 4, 5, 6). In Kraków region incidence was observed to be higher in urban than in rural populations [91].

Breast cancer risk higher in urban than in rural populations was also observed in other countries, but the urban preponderance there was not as large, the U/R ratio range being 1.2–1.3 : 1 [14,41,118].

The regional differences in breast cancer mortality in Poland in 1961 and the subsequent changes have been presented in other papers [173,176]. In 1961, mortality was highest in the five metropolitan cities, lead by Poznań City, and in Poznań, Katowice and Gdańsk districts. It was lowest in eastern districts, and in Koszalin and Szczecin districts [173]. The increase of breast cancer mortality in subsequent

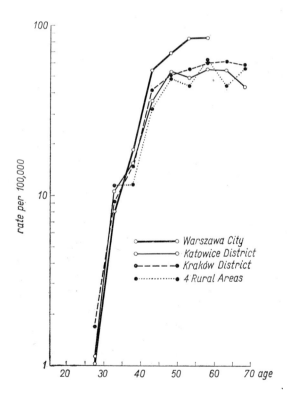

Fig. 8-4. Age-specific breast cancer incidence rates, per 100,000 females, in 1965–66 in the four regions of Poland.

years was greatest in the eastern and southern districts, where over-all cancer mortality was lowest in 1961 [170] and increased most in subsequent years. As a result, the range between the highest and lowest values narrowed appreciably, from 6 : 1 in 1961 to 2.75 : 1 in 1967–69, but the rank order of districts with respect to breast cancer mortality values was not much changed (Appendix Table 18, Figure 8-5).

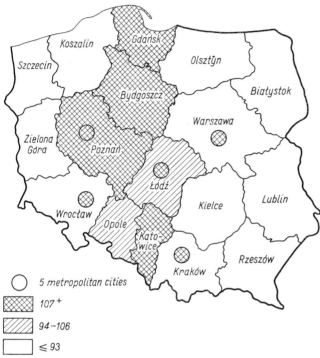

Fig. 8-5. Standardized mortality ratios, SMR, for breast cancer in females, by district of residence in 1967–69 in Poland. SMR = 100 for the total Polish population of the same sex and in the same period.

8.5. Time Trends

A small increase in breast cancer mortality, not exceeding 25 percent, was observed between 1950–1965 * in almost one-half of the 24 countries for which data were compiled by Segi et al. [160,161] — Finland, West Germany, Austria, Italy, Portugal, France, Belgium, Ireland, South Africa, Israel and Chile; in the remaining countries the mortality level did not change (Figure 8-7). Among white Americans and in England breast cancer mortality has not changed since 1930 [47,157], although it has increased by approximately 10 percent for the age groups under 55. In Connecticut breast cancer incidence increased by about 45 percent in the age groups under 55

* For Belgium that period was 1954–1965, and for Portugal 1956–1965, because the cited sources contain no earlier data for these countries.

in the 1930–1965 period, but did not change for older age groups [35]. In Norway breast cancer incidence increased by 15 percent in the 1955–1967 period; this trend was observed in all age groups [195].

Viewed in this context, the changes in Poland are striking. Analysing breast cancer mortality in Poland for the period 1952–1967, we have found that the

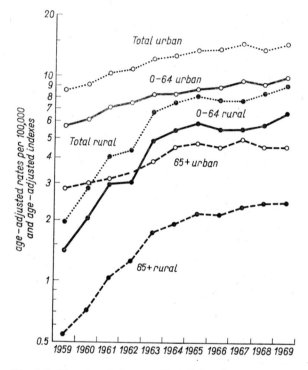

Fig. 8-6. Time trends in age-adjusted female breast cancer mortality rates and "age-adjusted indexes" up to and over 65 years of age, by urban-rural residence in the 1959–1969 period in Poland.

age-adjusted rates increased from 4.2 to 11.3 per 100,000 females or by 169 percent [176]. This increase was small between 1952–1959, only 22 percent, but great between 1959–1963 and greater in rural than in urban populations. It continued at a slower rate until 1969 (Figure 8-6). The fact that this increase was observed in all ages, both under and over 65, indicates that it was, at least partly, a true increase and not only the result of improved diagnosis.

In 1970 and 1971 a slow increase in breast cancer mortality rates in Poland continued (Figure 4-16).

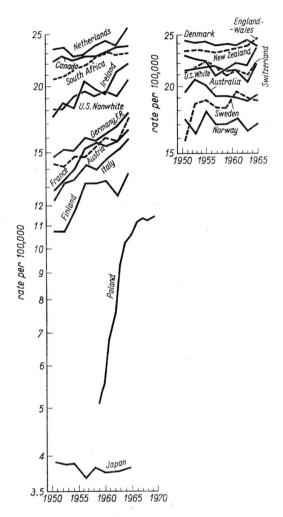

Fig. 8-7. Time trends in age-adjusted breast cancer mortality rates, per 100,000 females, in the 1950–1965 period as reported by Segi et al.[160,161] and in the 1959–1969 period in Poland.

8.6. Polish Migrants

Between 1950 and 1959–61, the breast cancer mortality of Polish-born Americans increased by only a few percent in each age group, whereas on the whole it did not change at all for white Americans[47]. The mortality rate of Polish-born Americans was much higher in all age groups than it was at the same time in Poland, even higher than present Polish rates, despite Poland's substantial increase in breast cancer mortality in recent years (Figure 8-8).

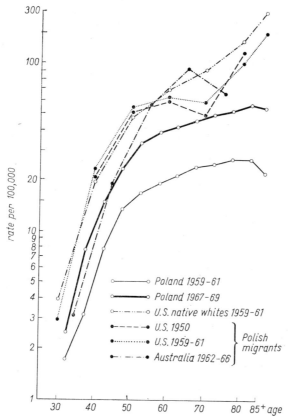

Fig. 8-8. Age-specific breast cancer mortality rates, per 100,000 females, in Poland, in Polish migrants to the United States and to Australia, and in native white Americans.

For younger females, up to the age group 45–54, the breast cancer mortality rate of Polish migrants was similar to that of native white Americans, but in the older age groups it was somewhat between the high mortality observed for native Americans and the low mortality prevailing in Poland. A similar incomplete transition to the high breast cancer mortality level in older age groups was observed only among Japanese and Italian migrants. It was not observed among migrants from five other European countries: England and Wales, Ireland, Sweden, Norway and Germany [60].

The behavior of the two segments of the mortality-by-age curve differed for the populations compared. The first segment, under age 55, was similar for Polish-born and for native Americans, and its slope was similar to that observed for Poland. The second or postmenopausal segment, however, was steepest for native Americans; the slope of this segment for urban females in Poland for 1967–69 was similar to that observed for native Americans, but for rural females it was similar to that observed for Polish and Italian migrants to the United States.

Breast cancer mortality among Polish migrants to Australia was higher than in Poland, close to the rates observed in Polish-born Americans (Figure 8-8, Appendix Table 17).

8.7. Discussion

8.7.1. Two Types of Breast Cancer

The bi-phasic relation of breast cancer occurrence to age is characteristic of this cancer (Figure 8-8). Up to about the age of 45, the rate of the increase with advancing age of breast cancer incidence and mortality is similar to that of most cancers, and shows little difference between high- and low-risk countries. For the older age groups, however, the rate of increase is slower; sometimes decrease of cancer occurrence with advancing age occurs; furthermore, the slope of this second segment of the age-curve varies between high- and low-risk populations. These observations led de Waard [203,204] to conclude that there are 2 types of breast cancer. One, which I shall call **type A**, seems to occur mainly before menopause and to depend on ovarian estrogens, whereas the other, **type B**, appears to occur mainly after menopause, to be related to obesity, hypertension and diabetes and to depend on corticosteroid production disturbances. Existence of two types of breast cancer, or of two types of its etiopathogenesis, has also been suggested by other authors [72,204].

If the existence of these two types of breast cancer is assumed, then type A would be prevalent in Japan, and type B in the western countries. The frequency of type B would be stable in the United States, whereas type A would be on the increase (see page 97). Subtracting the Japanese age-specific breast cancer mortality rates from the corresponding rates observed in western countries, de Waard obtained a new set of age-specific rates, which presumably represent the effect of the western environment and correspond to type B breast cancer. The rates thus obtained are represented on the log-log scale by straight, parallel lines, which are the higher in relation to the affluence of the respective country. According to Doll (see Chapter 4, Section 8), this linearity corresponds with a constant exposure to some carcinogenic factor, which acts with a different intensity in various countries. De Waard believes this factor to be overnutrition, which causes obesity and influences the hormonal pattern. Irrespective of what the nature of this factor may be, observations of Polish and Japanese migrants indicate either that its intensity increases slowly for these migrants, or that the manifestation of the effect of that increase on the type B appearance is delayed.

As to type A breast cancer, its incidence and mortality rates increase with age only up to the age of about 45 and decrease thereafter. It may be concluded that the factors responsible for this type also cease to act before that age. The risk of

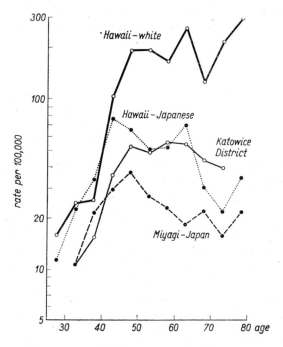

Fig. 8-9. Age-specific breast cancer incidence rates, per 100,000 females: A. Japan, Miyagi Prefecture, 1962–64; B. United States, Hawaii: Caucasian, 1960–64; C. United States, Hawaii: Japanese, 1960–64; D. Poland, Katowice District, 1965–66.

type A breast cancer increased among Polish migrants to the high level observed among native Americans, indicating that the intensity of the factors responsible for risk of type A had increased for these migrants and that the full effect of that increase became rapidly evident.

Morphological equivalents of the two postulated types of breast cancer are not yet known, but this does not prove they do not exist; existence of the two analogous types of stomach cancer has only recently been demonstrated (See page 54).

8.7.2. Factors Bearing on Breast Cancer Risk

There is a popular assumption that host factors, especially hormonal ones, play the most important role in etiopathogenesis of breast cancer. It is difficult, however, to interpret the significance and interrelation of genetic factors and acquired disposition related to environmental factors. (Hypotheses on the viral etiology of breast cancer will not be considered in the following discussion).

8.7.3. Genetic Factors

The significance of genetic factors in breast cancer etiopathogenesis has been demonstrated in experiments on animals; but some of the effect initially ascribed to inborn disposition was shown to be the result of other factors (Bittner's milk factor). It was also shown that observations made on one species cannot safely be generalized and transfered to other ones.

Unusually high incidences of breast cancer in some families suggest the importance of genetic factors in the etiopathogenesis of this neoplasm, but this phenomenon may be also ascribed to the similarity of environmental factors to which a given family is exposed.

Association between blood group A and breast cancer in young females (aged 40–44), suggested by Hems [72], requires corroboration.

Low breast cancer risk and especially its decrease in postmenopausal age groups, characteristic of Japan, is often believed to be caused by genetic factors [47]. Breast cancer incidence among Japanese migrants to the United States, however, shows a considerable increase (Figure 8-9).

According to the United States census of 1960, Japanese Americans living both in the continental United States and in Hawaii were characterized by the following interrelation between age and place of birth: most of those under 55 were members of the second generation (Nisei), but a predominate number of those in the older age groups had been born in Japan (Issei) [65]. From Figure 8-9 it can be seen that in 1960–64 breast cancer incidence among Nisei in Hawaii did not differ appreciably for those under the age of 45 from its incidence in whites. It seems that in the pre-menopausal age groups the migration effect on the Japanese was, at least in the second generation (Nisei), similar to that effect in the first generation of Polish and Italian migrants: displacement of type A breast cancer risk from the low level prevailing in the country of origin to the high level in the host country. In older age groups, especially those over 55 (in Issei) the migration effect was similar to that experienced by the first generation of Polish and Italian migrants to the United States: the risk of type B breast cancer was somewhere between that of the country of origin and that of the United States *.

These observations indicate the importance of environmental rather than genetic factors in breast cancer etiopathogenesis.

8.7.4. Acquired Disposition

Both laboratory and epidemiologic findings indicate the fundamental significance of hormonal factors, which are in turn dependent on such factors as parity

---

* It may be noted that the breast cancer incidence in Japanese migrants was similar to that in Poland, and was even higher in pre-menopausal age groups (Figure 8-9).

or nutrition. Bulbrook [23] found that breast cancer risk may be predicted by measuring proportions of some urinary steroids. He also tried to compare the endocrine function in British and Japanese women. Commenting on his findings, he states that: "... one striking difference between the populations was that the ratio of two of the androgen metabolites (androsterone and aetiocholanolone) is significantly higher in Japanese women after the menopause. This ratio is dependent on thyroid function and the present results indicate that Japanese women over the age of 40 have a greater thyroid function than that in British women... The next question was why thyroid function (as evidenced by the androgen metabolite ratio) should be increased in Japanese women. Dr. W. C. Mac Donald has been carrying out a study on the dietary habits of Japanese immigrants in Vancouver... Preliminary results indicate that the more Canadian food the immigrants eat, the nearer is the ratio of androsterone to aetiocholanolone to that found in British women. Immigrants still eating a typical Japanese diet have the high ratios found in Tokyo Japanese. The thesis that nutritional factors may affect endocrine function which in turn may affect the incidence of breast cancer may appear improbable but in the last few years some significant correlations have been found between the incidence of cancer and the amount of fat in the diet. Furthermore, mice fed on a Japanese type of diet show a reduced incidence of breast cancer" [23].

A relation between breast cancer risk and age at menarche was recently noticed [115,202,220]. Preliminary results of our investigations showed that in Poland females reporting menarche before the age of 16 have a breast cancer risk about 75 percent higher than those who began to menstruate at the age of 16 or over. In our material this relation between breast cancer risk and age at menarche was more distinct for patients under 45 than for older ones [179]. The percentage of females with a late menarche is much higher in Poland and Japan than it is in the United States. The decreasing percentage of females with a late menarche, observed in Poland [179] and in other countries [47,221], seems to be associated with an increase in breast cancer risk, especially of type A, as is suggested by the fact that the increase of breast cancer incidence in the United States is greater for females under 45. This probably is an indirect association, both the increasing breast cancer risk and the decreasing age at menarche being results of increasing affluence and improving nutrition.

Other explanations of the increased breast cancer risk of females with early menarche and of the increase in breast cancer incidence in premenopausal women are also possible. "With the earlier initiation of ovarian function, these young women would be at a higher risk, at any specific age, of developing breast cancer than were their older sisters at the same age" [47]. Otherwise, susceptibility to the possibly carcinogenic hormonal stimuli connected with menarche, might decrease with age. It is also conceivable that the speed of maturation is higher in girls with an early menarche than in those with a late one, and that the speed of maturation and specifically the increased speed of hormonal change and of breast tissue growth, might be the factor favoring breast cancer development.

The decreasing age at menarche, observed in Poland and in other countries, is ascribed to increasing affluence and improving nutrition [193]. Present knowledge is not sufficient to tell whether these factors mainly act just before menarche or at some earlier age [207,221].

An association between environmental conditions and nutrition on the one hand, and breast cancer occurrence on the other, has also been demonstrated.

Positive correlation of breast cancer rates with a high intake of animal protein [153], fat [25,72,208] and sugar [72] has been reported. According to Hems [72], the correlation with fat and sugar intake was closer for females aged 65–69 than for the 40–44 age-group.

Similarities between the epidemiologic characteristics of cancer of the breast (and of corpus uteri and ovarian cancer) and cancer of the intestinal tract [49,154,156] also suggest that dietary habits may have a bearing on the risk of these neoplasms.

Breast cancer risk increases with rising socioeconomic class. This relationship is distinct in Denmark [29] and even more distinct in Great Britain [191,197], but in the United States it seems to pertain only to immigrants [60].

Another characteristic noted among migrants to the United States, but not yet explained, is the distinct notch in the curve of breast cancer occurrence by age, similar to that described by Clemmesen for Denmark and observed subsequently in England and Norway, but absent among native white Americans [60].

Breast cancer risk is higher among nuns, unmarried [86,189,191] and nulliparous females [110,115]. This relationship seems to be confined to postmenopausal females [29,49]. The data routinely collected from the Oncological Institute in Gliwice, however, show that the percentage of nulliparous women in each age-group was higher in the 2744 breast cancer patients than in the 6949 women who made up the control group. In both groups the percentage of nulliparous women decreased with increasing age, up to about the age of 35 and did not change thereafter [185].

Decreased breast cancer risk has been observed among females reporting early first pregnancy (before the age of 20–25) and in females who have borne many children [149,202,220]. Among the 2744 breast cancer patients under study at the Oncological Institute in Gliwice, the percentage of women reporting seven or more parturitions was lower in all age groups than in the control group; this percentage had been decreasing for at least 20 years preceding collection of the data [185].

To summarize, it appears that in the last decade in Poland (at least in Silesia) the percentage of nulliparous women did not change, but the percentage of females bearing seven or more children (and this percentage is higher for rural than for urban females) had decreased greatly, a situation which might partly explain the increase in breast cancer mortality. The negative correlation between fertility distribution and breast cancer mortality also suggests that breast cancer risk depends on fertility. In western and northern districts, characterized by high fertility (Appendix Figure 2) and a high frequency of early marriages, this correlation differs from the one observed in other districts of Poland [173].

The negative association between breast feeding and breast cancer risk, previously assumed, is uncertain [115,149,211].

Surgical menopause prior to the age of 40 decreases breast cancer risk [46,77].

8.7.5. Interpretation

The observations presented above show the primary importance of hormonal factors in breast cancer etiopathogenesis. These hormonal factors, moreover, seem to be dependent on socioeconomic level and nutrition as well as on childbirths and, perhaps, under some circumstances, on breast feeding. Nutrition and socioeconomic level, which influence age at menarche, as well as childbirths, seem to have a bearing on breast cancer risk, and, combined, they may explain many of the differences and changes observed in the frequency of breast cancer occurrence. For example, this frequency, even for single or childless women, is much lower in Japan than in the United States [211] and may be related to the high proportion of women with a late menarche in Japan. The increase of breast cancer risk associated with the migration of Polish females to the United States does not seem to be connected with a change of age at menarche; nor does it appear to be associated with an increase of the percentage of single or childless women *. It is difficult to tell, however, if and to what extent the percentage of females bearing many children decreased or the quality of nutrition improved among Polish migrants; it is likely that the one or the other of these changes might possibly be the reason for the increase of breast cancer risk among these migrants. It is also possible that the very low proportion of single and childless women was partly responsible for the incomplete transition of the risk of postmenopausal (type B) breast cancer, among Polish and Italian migrants, to the high level prevailing in the United States. Such an assumption is supported by the observation that type B breast cancer was more frequent in Irish-born Americans than either in Ireland or among native-born Americans, and as many as 19.9 percent of the Irish-born were single and 15.7 percent of the married ones were childless [60].

Observations presented above indicate that, with respect to breast cancer, Poland is changing from a low-risk to a high-risk country and that the cities are leading in this process. This change is indicated not only by the increase of the mortality rates, but also by the increasing slope of the postmenopausal segment of the mortality-by-age curve. The low frequency of breast cancer occurrence in Poland, especially in rural populations, and its recent increase may be regarded,

---

* On the contrary, these percentages seem to have decreased in these migrants. The percentage of single (2.9) and of married childless females (6.0) was lower among Polish migrants in the United States, than among other major ethnic groups except Italians, whereas our data indicate that in Poland no less than 19 percent of females were childless [60,185].

on the basis of the available but still fragmentary data, as a result of improvements in both economic conditions and quality of nutrition (possibly in connection with the high but decreasing proportion of females with a late menarche), and also of the high, but decreasing frequency of numerous childbirth. Other factors such as the prevalence of breast feeding may also be involved in determining breast cancer risk.

Continuing study should help to determine the relative importance of such factors as age at menarche and at first childbirth or pregnancy, number of child-births, socioeconomic level and nutrition. The interrelation of such factors also requires investigation. For example, if protein deficiency results in decreasing breast cancer risk, then pregnancy and lactation should reduce this risk in low socio-economic classes but have little or no effect on females who eat well. In studying these factors, pre- and postmenopausal breast cancer cases should be separated. The time periods in which such factors as economic status or nutrition have changed, should also be ascertained. These time periods can be estimated in Po-land on the basis of the age of the person in question at the time of the First or Second World Wars. A combination of epidemiologic, pathomorphologic, hormonal and clinical studies might lead to determining whether there is a correlation bet-ween the epidemiologic type of breast cancer and its morphology or a patient's hormonal profile, whether the differences and changes in breast cancer occurrence have perceptible equivalents in hormonal differences between populations or in the occurrence of possibly precancerous lesions such as cystic hyperplasia among others.

Recently discovered similarities in the occurrence of breast cancer in humans and in dogs [155] indicate the desirability of comparative epidemiologic studies.

9 | Uterine Cancer

9.1. Opening Remarks

In 1967–69 uterus cancer caused 15.4 percent of all female cancer deaths and was second only to stomach cancer as a cause of cancer death in females.

A little more than half of all uterus cancer deaths were certified as the result of cervical cancer and only 12 percent as the result of corpus uteri cancer; over a third were classified as uterus cancer with no more detailed localization. Such a large proportion of tumors of unspecified uterine location makes it necessary to consider cancers of the uterine cervix and corpus jointly in the analysis of Polish mortality statistics. The following discussion will be limited almost entirely to uterus carcinomas because sarcomas and (in Europe) chorionepitheliomas constitute only a very small fraction of uterus cancers.

Cancer registration offers more detailed information on cancer localization in the uterus. In 1965–66, in the four selected regions of Poland, the age-adjusted incidence rate for cervical cancer accounted for 78–81 percent of the total uterus cancer incidence rate (69 percent in Rural Areas); the rates for corporal cancer accounted for 12–21 percent, and for the other and unspecified localization (Nos. 173 and 174, *ICD*, 1955 revision) for 4–10 percent. These data demonstrate that, in Polish mortality statistics, cervix uteri was the most frequent primary localization of tumors classified as "uterus, unspecified".

Cancer of the uterine cervix was the most frequent female cancer in all four Polish cancer registries.

Because of the high and still increasing curability of uterus cancer, morbidity statistics provide an independent and advantageous source of information about incidence since they are not distorted by the regional and secular variation in treatment results. Estimates of regional differences of the uterus cancer occurrence, however, based on both morbidity and mortality statistics, give similar and consistent results [53].

Temporary distortions resulting from mass screenings [131] and the lack of comparability of data from the registries, some of which include and some of which exclude the *in situ* carcinoma, are the main shortcomings of the uterus cancer morbidity statistics. For example, carcinoma *in situ* was reported as about 2 percent of all cervical cancers in the Kraków Register, about 6 percent in Katowice and in Colombia [41], about 30 percent in Warszawa [52], 33 percent in Norway, close to 50 percent in Sweden, and over 50 percent in Canada and in Connecticut [41].

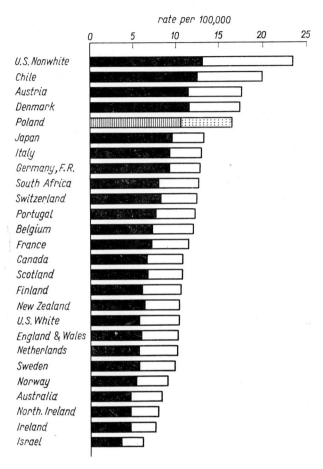

Fig. 9-1. Age-adjusted uterus cancer (Nos. 171–174, *ICD*, 1955 rev.) mortality rates, per 100,000 females, in 1964–65 in 24 countries [161] and in Poland. Shaded areas represent mortality under the age of 65.

9.2. Poland and Other Countries

Uterus cancer mortality in Poland would rank fifth among the 24 countries surveyed in 1964–65, after nonwhite Americans, Chile, Austria and Denmark (Figure 9-1). Cancer registration data [41] indicate that the incidence of cervix uteri cancer in Poland is rather high, although corpus uteri cancer incidence is low.

9 Epidemiology...

9.3. Age

Morbidity data will be considered first, because, as stated above, separation of cervical and corporal uterus cancer is incomplete in Polish mortality statistics.

Cervix uteri cancer is not rare among women even before the age of 30. The incidence of this cancer increased with age in all the four selected regions of Poland up to the age of 45, and remained on this level at older ages or even decreased slightly. Corpus uteri carcinoma, on the other hand, is rare before 40 and the increase of its incidence with age ceases first about 55–60 (Figure 9-2, Appendix Tables 3, 4, 5, 6).

Cancer registration data [41] indicate that the shape and slope of the incidence-by--age curve for both cervical and corporal uterus cancer in Poland are similar to those plotted for other countries.

The difference in the relationship of both these cancers to age causes their proportions to vary with age. Data from the four selected regions of Poland [41] show that cervical cancer accounts for more than 80 percent of all uterus cancers in wo-

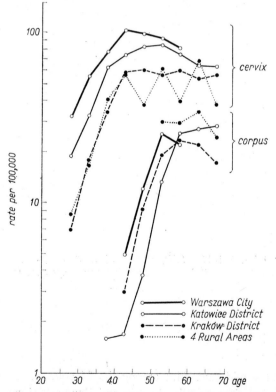

Fig. 9-2. Age-specific uterine cervix cancer (No. 171) and uterine corpus cancer (No. 174, *ICD*, 1955 rev.) incidence rates, per 100,000 females, in 1965–66 in the four regions of Poland.

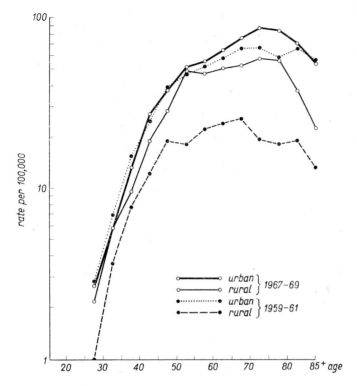

Fig. 9-3. Age-specific uterus cancer (Nos. 171–174, *ICD*, 1955 rev.) mortality rates, per 100,000 females, by urban-rural residence in 1959–61 and 1967–69 in Poland.

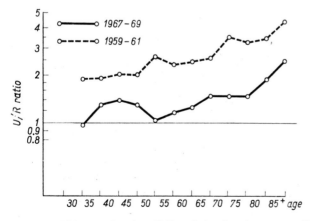

Fig. 9-4. Urban-rural ratios, U/R, of the female age specific uterus cancer (Nos. 171–174, *ICD*, 1955 rev.) mortality rates in 1959–61 and 1967–69 in Poland.

men under 55. At older ages this percentage decreases to about 65 and the percentage of cancer of the corpus increases to about 25; more detailed localization of the remaining 10 percent of uterus cancers is unspecified. We may conclude that Polish mortality statistics on uterus cancer depict cervical cancer mortality well in women under 55, but not so well for the older age groups; this same conclusion may be drawn from a comparison of cervix and corpus cancer incidence with the incidence of uterus cancer as a whole (Figures 9-2 and 9-5).

The increase with age of uterus cancer mortality rates in Poland slows down among women over 50, somewhat later than the slowdown in incidence rates for cervix uteri cancer and less conspicuous (Figure 9-3).

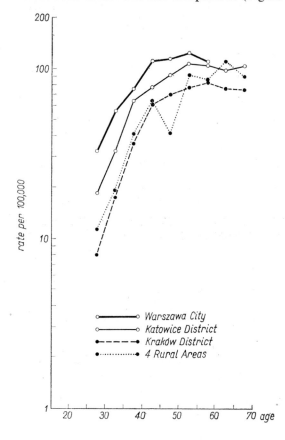

Fig. 9-5. Age-specific uterus cancer (Nos. 171–174, *ICD*, 1955 rev.) incidence rates, per 100,000 females, in the four regions of Poland.

9.4. Residence

The urban-rural ratio of the uterus cancer mortality rates, U/R, in Poland decreased from 2.39 : 1 in 1959–61 to 1.28 : 1 in 1967–69. This decrease occurred in all age groups. The U/R ratio is now only slightly above 1 : 1 for females under 60, but for older females it increases with advancing age (Figures 9-3 and 9-4).

Analysis of regional differences in uterus cancer mortality in Poland in 1961 revealed that the highest mortality rates were in the western and northern districts (including Katowice and Opole Districts); of the 5 metropolitan cities, Wrocław had the highest mortality rates, and Kraków and Warszawa the lowest [184]. This pattern had not changed much in 1967–69 (Figure 9-6, Appendix Table 18).

For all age groups, the cervix uteri cancer incidence rates, taken at their face values, show the highest incidence in Warszawa City, intermediate incidence in Katowice District, and lowest incidence in Kraków Region and in Rural Areas (Figure 9-2). But if the incidence of *in situ* carcinoma, which accounted for about 30 percent of cervix uteri cancer in Warszawa City register [52] but was not included in the Katowice and Kraków rates, were excluded from the comparison, the incidence rates of invasive cervical cancer for Warszawa City would be somewhat lower than those for Katowice District.

9.5. Time Trends

In the 1950–1965 period uterus cancer mortality rates decreased distinctly in 16 out of 24 countries, including Australia and the United States (both white and nonwhite females) (Figure 9-8). In the remaining eight countries, including Chile and Denmark, they maintained the same level, often with some downward tendency. Information from cancer registries, however, indicates that the incidence level for both invasive cervical and corporal cancer remains relatively unchanged [14,29] or even shows some increase [195]. It therefore seems that the decrease in uterus cancer mortality observed in many countries was primarily the result of improved treatment.

In this context the increase in uterus cancer mortality rates in Poland in the 1959–1969 period is striking (Figure 9-7). This increase continued only until 1963 or 1964 and although considerable in the rural population, especially for older age groups, it was only slight in the urban population for females aged 65 and over, and either nonexistant or negative for women under 50. These observations will be discussed below in Discussion.

9.6. Polish Migrants

Uterus cancer mortality rates among Polish-born Americans in 1959–61 were lower than they were in Poland in the age groups under 60, and higher in the older ones; they were also somewhat lower than among native white Americans (Figure 9-9). Mortality among Polish born Americans in all age groups below 70 decreased greatly in comparison to the 1950 rates; the age-adjusted rates decreased by one third, as they did among native white Americans in the same time period.

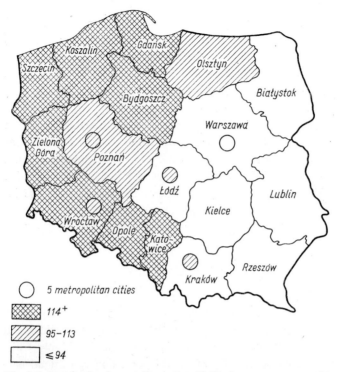

Fig. 9-6. Standardized mortality ratios, SMR, for uterus cancer (Nos. 171–174, *ICD*, 1955 rev.) in females, by district of residence in 1967–69 in Poland. SMR = 100 for the total Polish population of the same sex and in the same period.

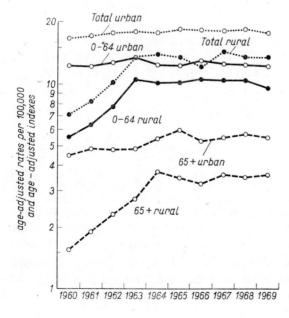

Fig. 9––7. Time trends in age-adjusted female uterus cancer (Nos. 171–174, *ICD*, 1955 rev.) mortality rates and "age-adjusted indexes" up to and over 65 years of age, by urban-rural residence in the 1959–1969 period in Poland.

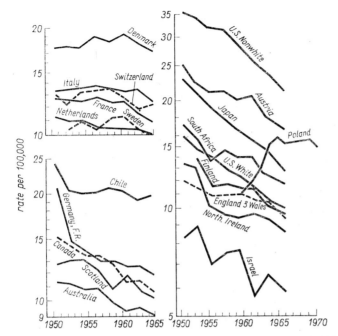

Fig. 9-8. Time trends in age-adjusted uterus cancer (Nos. 171–174, *ICD*, 1955 rev.) mortality rates, per 100,000 females, in the 1950–65 period as reported by Segi et al. [160,161] and in the 1959–1969 period in Poland.

In 1950 [180], as well as in 1959–61, mortality rates for both cervical and corporal uterus cancer were similar among Polish-born and native white Americans. This indicates that the cervical cancer risk among Polish migrants was displaced downwards from the high level characteristic of Poland to the lower one observed among native white Americans, whereas the risk of uterine corpus cancer among these migrants rose to a level higher than the low one prevailing in their country of origin. A similar differential in the displacement of cervix and corpus uteri mortality was observed in Japanese migrants to the United States [65].

There were only 17 deaths ascribed to uterus cancer among Polish migrants to Australia: 11 of the cervix, 4 of the corpus, and 2 unspecified. These numbers are too small to permit conclusions regarding migration effects.

9.7. Discussion

9.7.1. Uterus Cancer

The incomplete separation of cervical and corporal uterus cancer in Polish mortality statistics compels us to consider them jointly although contrasting epidemiologic characteristics indicate the desirability of separating these two cancers in

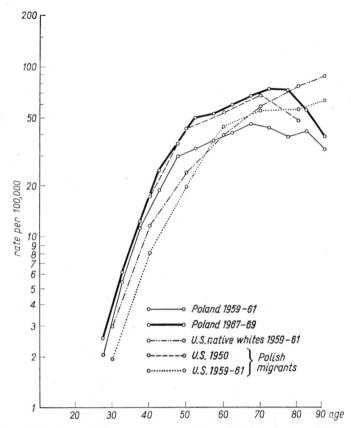

Fig. 9-9. Age-specific uterus cancer (Nos. 171–174, *ICD*, 1955 rev.) mortality rates, per 100,000 females, in Poland, in Polish-migrants to the United States and in native white Americans.

epidemiologic studies. When cervical cancer distinctly predominates, as it does in Poland, uterus cancer mortality may reflect cervical cancer mortality and risk fairly well. This is true especially for the age groups up to about 55; for older age groups such estimates of cervical cancer occurrence are less and less accurate.

Any comparison of the regional distribution and time trends of cervical cancer occurrence in Poland with age at first coitus, number of partners, number of pregnancies or parturitions or with other factors suspected of having some bearing on the risk of this cancer, is impossible because of the lack of necessary data. Using mortality statistics, however, it was possible to compare uterus cancer occurrence by district with the distribution of fertility rates and the proportions of married persons in the young age groups; the relationship between these factors and cervical cancer is, of course, partly obscured by the corporal cancer component, which distorts these comparisons. When the metropolitan cities, and the Katowice and Opole Districts, where both fertility rates and the proportion of early marriages were low but uterus cancer mortality was high, were eliminated from the comparison, marked correlation between these factors and uterus cancer mortality was demonstrated [184]. Such a correlation would probably be even more marked if comparisons were limited only to cervical cancer: the proportion of corporal cancer is probably higher, in metropolitan cities at least, than it is in other districts; this situation is indicated by the high standardized indexes for the ages of 65 and over found for these cities, an observation which demonstrates that metropolitan cities display higher uterus cancer mortality rates than the other districts for the age groups in which corporal cancer proportion is substantial. The relatively high rate of uterus cancer mortality in Katowice, Opole and Gdańsk Districts is consistent with reports from other countries that cervical cancer risk is greater in industrial areas and seaports [190].

In most countries and populations, including Polish-born Americans, a decrease in uterus cancer mortality is apparent, primarily the result of more frequent early detection and increasing curability of this cancer. In contrast to this, uterus cancer mortality increased in Poland in the 1959–1969 period. This increase, however, divides into several components. A rapid increase in mortality rates took place among both urban and rural females 65 and over and a less rapid increase among younger rural, but not urban females prior to 1964. This increase appears to have been primarily the result of improved diagnosis rather than of an actual increase in the disease. Since 1964 uterus cancer mortality in Poland has remained at the same level (Figure 9-7).

The increase in the frequency of corpus uteri cancer is indicated by the increase in the slope of the mortality-by-age curve observed for females over 55.

The present slight decrease in uterus cancer mortality among younger urban females indicates that cervical cancer mortality may be decreasing in Poland, at least in urban areas.

9.7.2. Corpus Uteri Cancer

Hyperestrogenism is believed to be an important factor in the etiopathogenesis of this cancer. The high corporal cancer risk of women with feminizing ovarial tumors, for example, is well known.

Corporal cancer displays epidemiologic similarities to breast cancer, especially to type B (postmenopausal). Increased corporal cancer risk has been demonstrated for females with breast cancer, and increased breast cancer risk for females with corporal cancer, especially for those over 60 [13,114]. Both cancers are more frequent among single, childless females, and in higher socioeconomic classes. Both are associated with obesity, hypertension, diabetes, infertility [203,208,212], intestinal tract cancer [154,156], and with the high consumption of animal proteins [150,153] and fats [208,212].

Information about corporal cancer geography is less complete than about breast cancer, but it points to similarities between these two cancers. They occur most frequently in North America, Western Europe, and the Scandinavian countries, and less frequently in Japan and in Poland. Among migrants to the United States mortality rates for both these cancers increased more for Polish than for Japanese females.

9.7.3. Cervix Uteri Cancer

Epidemiologic studies have provided much information, shedding light on the etiopathogenesis of this cancer. Mass screenings have helped to collect knowledge about the lesions which precede the appearance of the invasive carcinoma in the uterine cervix [44,81]. Much information about factors associated with this neoplasm has also been collected.

Genetic factors are probably not of primary importance for cervical cancer; familial aggregations of this neoplasm have not been ascertained [143,144]; and claims that it is associated with some blood groups are uncertain [80,122,145]. The rarity of cervical cancer among Jewish females seems to depend on environmental factors, possibly including the Jewish practice of circumcision, rather than on the genetic ones.

Cervical cancer is infrequent in populations in which the frequency of penis cancer is low and circumcision is common, but case-control studies have cast some doubt on the association between circumcision and decreased cervical cancer risk [1,4]. A negative correlation between socioeconomic class and level of hygiene has been demonstrated for both cancer of the uterine cervix and of the penis [54,87,164,190,197]. The high frequency of cervical cancer in Poland, however, is not associated with a high frequency of penis cancer [41,100]. Cervical cancer risk is greater for married females [110,189], especially for those who married early or more than once, for those who have borne many children or have had many abortions, and for those who began their sexual lives early and have had many partners [142,164]. The interdependence of these factors makes it difficult to ascertain which of them are most important and which are only indirectly associated with cervical cancer. For example, the significance of childbearing and gravidity is still uncertain. Puerperal trauma to the uterine cervix was formerly thought to be an important risk factor, but the association between parturition and cervical cancer is now believed to be rather secondary, the important factor actually being sex life, including such elements as frequency of heterosexual intercourse, age at first coitus and, possibly, number of partners. This view is based on the results of studies carried out in the United States and in Great Britain [4,142,190]. The results of an ongoing case-control study in Poland [164], however, indicate that cervical cancer risk is dependent on the number of parturitions even after an adjustment has been made for age at first intercourse. Similar results were recently reported from India [205]. It would be interesting to discover the factors responsible for these differences between Poland and India on the one hand and the Western countries on the other, in the role of parturition in cervical cancer etiopathogenesis.

The nature of the association between sexual life and cervical cancer risk mentioned above is not yet known, but the accumulated epidemiologic observations not only permit the formulation of some interesting hypotheses, but also forecast the early emergence of a correct explanation.

The hypothesis that some chemical carcinogen, possibly contained in smegma, is crucial for the etiopathogenesis of cervical cancer, is supported by the association known to exist between this cancer and hygiene and circumcision. The fact that the occurrence of cervical cancer seems to be only slightly related to frequency of coitus argues against this hypothesis as does the fact that this cancer also appears among females who had a few or even only one coitus [142,164].

On the contrary, these observations support the hypothesis that viral infection causes cervical cancer. This hypothesis is further corroborated by the demonstration of the appearance, more frequently in cervical cancer patients than in controls, of the antibodies to genital *Herpesvirus hominis*, Type 2 herpesvirus which, in contrast to Type 1, is most probably transmitted venereally and can produce lesions in the genital organs. These antibodies, absent from the serum of girls in their first decade of life, are present in an increasing proportion of girls in their second decade. The proportion of females possessing these antibodies does not increase, however, among those over 25; furthermore the proportion is negatively correlated with socioeconomic class [128,134]. Genital herpes occurs less frequently among circumcised than uncircumcised males [134]. The viral hypothesis is thus consistent with epidemiologic observations, but this circumstance alone does not prove a causal association, since cervical cancer may be caused by some other factor, related to sexual life in a way similar to the virus. The verification of the viral hypothesis would require combined case-control and virusologic studies. At the present time the infectious etiopathogenesis of cervical cancer seems quite likely even though *Herpesvirus* may not be its cause.

Reid's hypothesis [136,137] that the spermatozoa phaged by cervical mucosa cells may act as mutagens and cause cancerization of these cells, may be considered a variant of the infectious or viral hypothesis. Dependence of cervical cancer risk on the number of sexual partners suggests that only some males are carriers; this observation, as well as the association between cervical cancer and socioeconomic class and hygiene is more difficult to reconcile with Reid's hypothesis than with the viral hypothesis.

Most probably, the events leading to the development of cervical cancer, which may be parturitions, pregnancies or instances of sexual intercourse, take place, as a rule, between the ages of 15–45, and usually in the earlier years of this period. The "latency" interval between these events and clinical diagnosis of or death from cervical cancer is usually several decades. In Rotkin's study, for example, the interval between first coitus and the clinical appearance of cervical cancer was, on the average, 29 years, with a quite symmetric distribution [142]. In only 4.7 percent of the cases was this interval over 50 or under 11 years. The earlier first intercourse occurred the longer the interval before cancer appeared; on the average, it was 30–32 years for those who first experienced coitus before the age of 21, and 24–26 years for those whose first coitus occurred after the age of 23.

Too much emphasis is probably placed upon age at first intercourse. The observations presented above are easier to account for on the basis of the hypothesis that some venereally transmitted factor, possibly a virus, possibly spermatozoa, carry the infection, assuming further that the true latency interval between this infection and cancer appearance does not depend on age at which this factor acts.

If the hypothesis just proposed is true, age at first infectious coitus would determine only the moment at which cancer risk is initiated. It would be exactly equivalent to age at first coitus only for women who have no more than one partner (assuming in addition that each act of intercourse with the infectious partner is also infectious). Females who begin their sex lives late usually have fewer partners, a factor that may explain both their lower cervical cancer risk and that shorter latency interval which, on the average, would be closer to the true interval between infectious coitus to the appearance of cancer. On the other hand, females who begin their sex lives early seem to have more partners; the interval between first coitus and coitus with an infectious partner will, on the average, be longer so that the observable latency period which is measured from first coitus rather than from first infectious coitus (which cannot be determined) will also be longer. A larger number of partners increases the chance of encountering an infectious one and therefore increases cervical cancer risk.

10 | Prostate Cancer

10.1. Opening Remarks

In 1967–69, prostate cancer accounted for 5.4 percent of cancer deaths among men in Poland. In cancer registries in the selected regions of Poland in 1965–66, this tumor accounted for about 3.5 percent of the new cancer cases in Katowice and Kraków Districts, and about 6 percent in Warszawa City and in the Rural Areas.

It is not always easy to diagnose prostate cancer which appears primarily in the oldest age groups, where cancer diagnosis is the least accurate. Victims of prostate cancer often die from other causes, so that evaluation of its occurrence based on mortality statistics is less accurate than evaluation of the occurrence of cancers discussed in the preceding chapters. Difficulties resulting from the frequent occurrence of symptomless cancer in the prostatic gland will be discussed below, in section 10.7.1.

10.2. Poland and Other Countries

Compared with prostate cancer mortality in 24 countries in 1964–65, mortality in Poland would rank last but one (Figure 10-1). Morbidity statistics also indicate a low frequency of prostate cancer occurrence in Poland; cancer incidence reported by registries in the selected regions of Poland is lower than the incidence observed in other registries except those of Bombay and of Japan [41].

10.3. Age

The speed with which the incidence and mortality rates for prostate cancer increase with age is much greater than it is for any other cancer. Among males between 35 and 64 in most countries, including Poland, this increase is proportional to about the eleventh power of age, although for most other cancers it is proportional to the 4–7th powers of age [30,38].

The slope of the mortality-by-age curve in Poland in 1967–69 was similar to that of other countries, including the United States, Japan, Great Britain, and the Scandinavian countries. The shape of this curve varied only for the oldest age groups, for which the mortality increase with age slowed down more markedly in

Poland and Japan than in the other countries mentioned. This phenomenon was the result of a decrease in prostate cancer mortality rates in oldest age groups of the rural population, most probably caused by the decreasing, with advancing age, accuracy in diagnosis of cause of death. On the other hand, the mortality-by-age

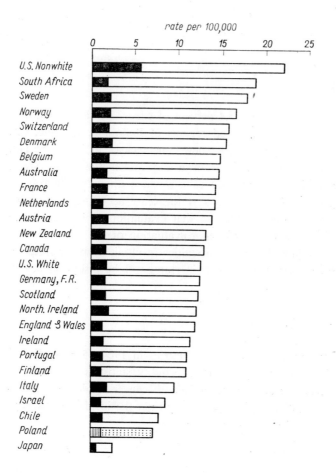

Fig. 10-1. Age-adjusted prostate cancer mortality rates, per 100,000 males, in 1964–65 in 24 countries [161] and in Poland. Shaded areas represent mortality under the age of 65.

curve for the urban Polish population was shaped like those of Western countries even for the oldest ages (Figure 10-2).

The essential difference between Poland and the Western countries with regard to the mortality-by-age curve for prostate cancer is in the position of that curve, placed more towards lower values of the mortality rate for all age groups although not so much as the curve for Japan.

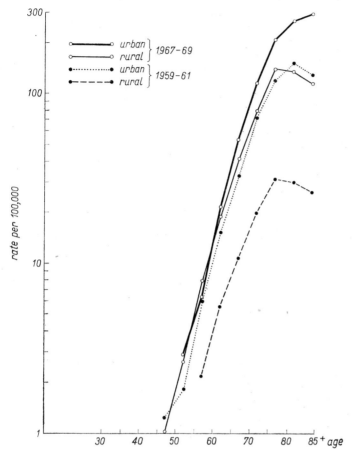

Fig. 10-2. Age-specific prostate cancer mortality rates, per 100,000 males, by urban-rural residence in 1959–61 and 1967–69 in Poland.

10.4. Residence

The urban-rural ratio, U/R, of the age-adjusted prostate cancer mortality rates in Poland decreased from 3.62 : 1 in 1959–61 to 1.49 : 1 in 1967–69. This decrease could be seen in all age groups over 55; the mortality rates among males under 55 were so low that the U/R ratio is unstable (Figure 10-3).

The U/R ratio observed currently in Poland is similar to that reported some-what earlier from other countries. For example, according to King et al. [84] the U/R ratio of the prostate cancer incidence rates was 1.1–1.2 : 1 in the United States, 1.5 : 1 in Denmark (where Copenhagen was compared with rural areas), 1.6 : 1 in Norway * and 2.0 : 1 in Finland; for mortality rates the U/R ratio in the United States was 1.3 : 1.

* According to more recent data, the U/R ratio in Norway is 1.25 : 1 [41].

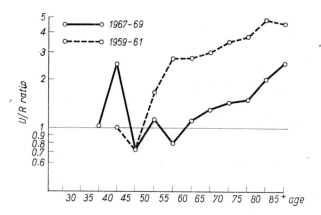

Fig. 10-3. Urban-rural ratios, U/R, of the male age-specific prostate cancer mortality rates in 1959–61 and 1967–69 in Poland.

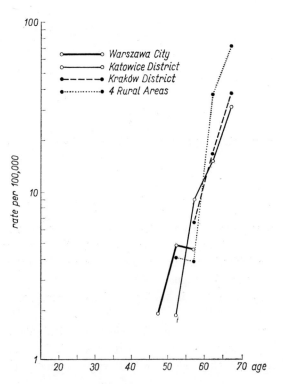

Fig. 10-4. Age-specific prostate cancer incidence rates, per 100,000 males, in 1965–66 in the four regions of Poland.

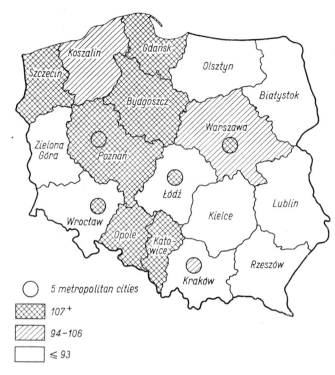

Fig. 10-5. Standardized mortality ratios, SMR, for prostate cancer in males, by district of residence in 1967–69 in Poland. SMR = 100 for the total Polish population of the same sex and in the same period.

5 metropolitan cities

107 +

94–106

≤ 93

Polish cancer registration data indicate that the incidence of prostate cancer is highest in Warszawa City. A more detailed comparison is impractical because the oldest age groups, in which most cases of prostate cancer are encountered, have not been subdivided (Figure 10-4, Appendix Tables 3-6).

For the same reason (see Chapter 3.3), the SMR's for cancer of the prostate presented in Appendix Table 18 and Figure 10-5 should be considered as tentative values only. They indicate that in 1967–69 prostate cancer mortality was highest in metropolitan cities (especially Poznań) and in Gdańsk, Poznań, Bydgoszcz, Katowice, Opole nad Szczecin Districts.

10.5. Time Trends

The age-adjusted prostate cancer mortality rates increased in the 1950–1965 period in most of the 24 countries, with the exception of the United States * and Australia (Figure 10-7). The rates increased by 20–50 percent, except in Japan where the

* In the United States prostate cancer incidence has probably increased, whereas mortality, especially for those under the age of 80, has decreased a little. The small increase in incidence seems to be balanced by improved prognosis [53].

increase was as high as 400 percent. The age-adjusted prostate cancer incidence rates in Norway increased in the 1955–1967 period by close to 20 percent [195]. The increase of nearly 300 percent in the prostate cancer mortality rates in Poland, observed in an 11-year period, is thus exceptionally high, comparable only to that of Japan.

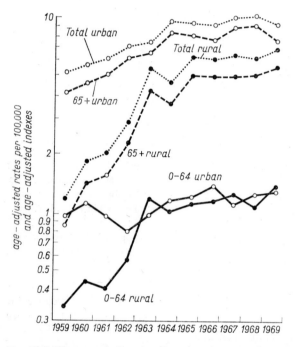

Fig. 10-6. Time trends in age-adjusted male prostate cancer mortality rates and "age-adjusted indexes" up to and over 65 years of age, by urban-rural residence in the 1959–1969 period in Poland.

The increase in the prostate cancer mortality rates in Poland was much greater for the rural than for the urban population (Figure 10-6). It was greatest up to 1964, and much less rapid thereafter. Since it involved all age groups and both urban and rural populations (albeit to a different extent), this increase appears to have been in part genuine and not solely the result of improved diagnosis.

The increase in prostate cancer mortality in Poland continued in 1970 and 1971 (Figure 4-15).

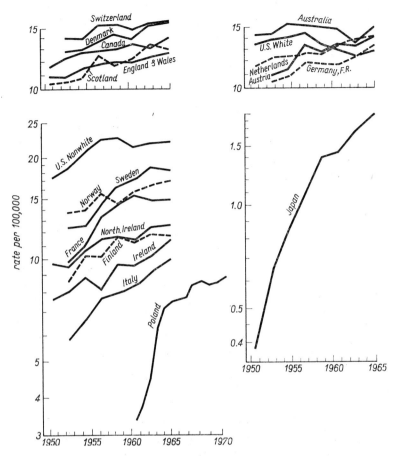

Fig. 10-7. Time trends in age-adjusted prostate cancer mortality rates, per 100,000 males, in the 1950–1965 period as reported by Segi et al. [160,161] and in the 1959–1969 period in Poland.

10.6. Polish Migrants

In 1959–1961, prostate cancer mortality among Polish-born Americans was about 3 times as high as in Poland, but about 20 percent lower than it was among native white Americans (Figure 10-8). In 1950, mortality among Polish-born Americans was also about 20 percent lower than among native white Americans and, presumably, much higher than in Poland. Increased prostate cancer mortality, likewise not reaching the high level experienced by native Americans, was also observed among migrants from other low-risk countries, including Japan, Italy, Czechoslovakia and the U.S.S.R. [60,65].

Since only eight deaths from prostate cancer were observed among Polish migrants to Australia, the number is too low to permit any conclusions.

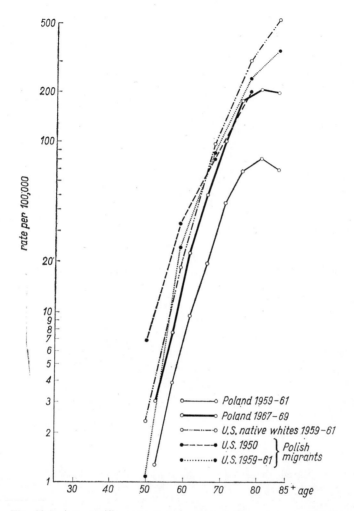

Fig. 10-8. Age-specific prostate cancer mortality rates, per 100,000 males, in Poland, in Polish migrants to the United States and in native white Americans.

10.7. Discussion

10.7.1. Symptomatic versus Asymptomatic Cancer

Evaluation of prostate cancer occurrence is difficult because of two specific features of this neoplasm:

1) most cases reported are in the oldest age groups;

2) necropsy studies of persons who died from other diseases indicate a very high frequency of cases of asymptomatic prostate cancer, as high as "... eighty-fold dif-

ference between the death rate for cancer of the prostate and the observed incidence of the tumor in unselected necropsy material, a discrepancy not observed in other tumor types" [9].

The first of these features decreases the accuracy of information on prostate cancer occurrence, because the accuracy in detecting cancer, as well as in determining causes of death, is lowest in the oldest age groups.

It is believed that, considering the high frequency of asymptomatic ("clinically latent") cases, mortality data have some advantages over morbidity statistics: "... high frequency of "clinically latent" cases may be expected to make incidence rates dependent on intensity with which post mortem examination is performed..." [29]. "Deaths certified to cancer of the prostate usually present clinical symptoms, and mortality data may be more easily compared than incidence data, which can include asymptomatic cases diagnosed by study of surgical and necropsy specimens" [65].

Epidemiologic differences between symptomatic and asymptomatic prostate cancer create further difficulties in studying the occurrence of this neoplasm. For example, although prostate cancer mortality in Western European countries and in the United States is several times as high as in Japan, the frequency of asymptomatic prostate cancer was found to be similar in Japan and in these countries. Akazaki speculates that the Japanese may be deficient in some endogenous factor that stimulates the proliferation and dedifferentiation of latent prostatic cancer cells [5,61]. Ashley even suggests that the clinically active and the clinically latent prostate cancers are two different biological entities. It appears from his estimates that the incidence of "latent" carcinoma of the prostate is proportional to the second or third power of age, which corresponds to a much lower slope in the curve of dependence on age than was established for symptomatic cancer of the prostate [9].

In a recent study, based on 500 consecutive autopsies [111], Luciak demonstrated a prevalence of the latent prostate cancer in Poland as high as in the Western countries — a finding contrasting with the apparently low frequency of occurrence of symptomatic prostate cancer in Poland (Table 10-1).

Table 10-1

	Percentage of autopsies with latent „occult" prostate cancer, reported by Luciak [111]						
	A g e						
	0–30	31–40	41–50	51–60	61–70	71–80	81–90
Number of autopsies studied	64	56	68	111	134	58	9
% of latent prostate cancers	0.0	1.8	4.4	7.2	14.3	17.2	44.4

Such observations indicate the need for separate consideration of the symptomatic and "latent" cases of prostate cancer. The two variants will be difficult to separate, especially in cancer registries; but if they are not separated, different sources of information may begin to provide contradictory estimates of the occurrence of prostate cancer. In the following discussion only symptomatic cancer will be considered, unless otherwise specified.

Little is yet known of the factors bearing on prostate cancer risk.

10.7.2. Genetic Factors

These factors might account for the high frequency of this cancer among male relatives of prostate cancer decedents [84]. Displacements in risk of this cancer observed in migrant populations, however, indicate that environmental factors are of greater importance in the etiopathogenesis of this neoplasm.

10.7.3. Nutrition

It has been suggested that prostate cancer risk increases with increasing consumption of animal proteins [151] or animal fats [209]. This relationship might account for the negative correlation between prostate cancer and cancer of the stomach, such as the low frequency of prostate cancer and high frequency of stomach cancer in Japan, Chile, and Poland; and for the positive correlation with intestinal tract and breast cancer both of which are relatively rare in those countries. Taking into consideration the speculations of Akazaki mentioned above, one can further conjecture that dietary deficiencies in animal proteins or fats impede the transformation of latent prostate cancer into symptomatic cancer. This dietary factor might either have a direct effect on the prostate or act indirectly by changing the hormonal status.

The low frequency of prostate cancer observed in Poland and its increase, corresponding to the increase in protein and fat consumption, as shown in Appendix Figure 1, is consistent with the hypothesis that development of this cancer depends on nutrition. This hypothesis may also account for the increase in the prostate cancer risk observed among Polish migrants to the United States. This increase indicates that factors acting in the later periods of life are more important in the development of this cancer than in the development of stomach cancer. Such an explanation is consistent with the assumption that dietary deficiencies may damage the stomach mucosa during childhood and favor the development of stomach cancer (see Chapter 5.8); whereas in adulthood these deficiencies may prevent either the development of prostate cancer or transformation of latent into symptomatic cancer. However, some observations can hardly be accounted for by these hypotheses, which indicates that some other factors may also be important in the prostate cancer etiopathogenesis.

10.7.4 Factors Related to Sex Life and Hygiene

The age-adjusted prostate cancer mortality rates for males who have ever been married are higher than the rates for those who remained single [84]. Clemmesen [29] noted that this disparity does not include the younger age groups, and that this cancer is even somewhat more frequent in single than in ever-married males under the age of 55. He directs attention to, but does not comment upon, the similarity of this phenomenon to the reversal in the single-to-married ratio observed for female breast cancer.

Similarities in geographic occurrence between cancers of the prostate and breast were mentioned above. The two most conspicuous exceptions to this correlation are Israel, where prostate cancer is less frequent than would be expected on the basis of breast cancer frequency, and the United States among non-whites, for whom very high prostate cancer mortality rates are reported, about three times as high as the rates for white Americans in most age groups.

The low frequency of prostate cancer in Jews is ascribed to circumcision [6], and therefore may be related to hygiene. Such a conclusion is further supported by the apparent association of this cancer with prostatitis [209]. Some similarities in the epidemiology of cancer of the prostate and of the uterine cervix, such as their decreased risk in single persons, may also be relevant. Although parallel occurrence patterns of these two cancers can be noted (both are frequent among black Americans and infrequent among Jews), contrasts in their occurrence can also be found, such as the high frequency of cervical cancer accompanied by a low frequency of prostate cancer in Chile, Japan, and Poland or the opposite situation, found among Irish migrants to the United States.

These observations suggest that the development of prostate cancer may be dependent on two groups of factors:

1) dietary habits and nutrition, or hormonal factors dependent on nutrition, which would account for the epidemiologic similarities to cancer of the breast and of the uterine corpus;

2) factors related to hygiene and sex life, accounting for similarities with uterine cervix cancer occurrence.

The effects of these two groups of factors may cancel one another, accounting for the lack of association between prostate cancer and socioeconomic class [84], although uterine cervix cancer risk is highest in the lower socioeconomic classes and the breast cancer risk in the upper classes.

11 | Final Remarks and Conclusions

11.1. Cancer Occurrence in Poland and in Polish Migrants, and Hypotheses on the Etiopathogenesis of Cancer

The purpose of this section is to recall how the observations presented in the preceding chapters are related to knowledge of and hypotheses about the etiopathogenesis of the cancers discussed.

11.1.1. Cancer of the Stomach and of the Intestinal Tract

Dietary habits and nutrition seem to be among the most important factors determining the risk of these cancers. Little is yet known whether or to what extent locally acting carcinogens, present in food or formed in the lumen of the alimentary canal, or factors which influence the contact of carcinogens with mucosa, or dietary deficiencies are involved. There is also a possibility that the co-carcinogenic action of other factors, such as tobacco smoking in the development of cancer of some stomach parts, is involved.

The high, but decreasing risk of stomach cancer in Poland, as well as its distinct negative correlation with socioeconomic class, is consistent with the hypothesis that dietary deficiencies are important for development of this neoplasm. The same observations, however, can also be accounted for by the hypothesis that the type of diet predominating in Poland until recent years contained carcinogens, possibly produced by microorganisms during the fermentation or storage of food, while post-war changes in dietary habits reduced exposure to these carcinogens.

The low but increasing incidence of colorectal cancer observed in Poland is consistent with the view that the risk of these neoplasms is increased among populations in which consumption of fats, sugar and meat is high; but it is difficult to draw more specific conclusions about the etiopathogenesis of these cancers from such observations.

The frequency of stomach cancer occurrence is usually high in those populations in which intestinal tract cancer frequency is low, and vice versa. Such a negative correlation is noticeable in Poland, in the United States and in Japan, but not among Polish migrants. Changes in the risk of these cancers, occurring in migrant populations, differ thus not only in direction, but also over time; the increase in the frequency of intestinal tract cancer is apparent much more promptly than the decrease in stomach cancer frequency. Therefore, it is probable that the determining factors for cancer risk are different for various parts of the alimentary canal. It is also possible, however, that the time it takes for the negative effect of such factors (i.e. increased risk of the intestinal tract cancer) to materialize is shorter than the time it takes for their positive effect (i.e. decreased stomach cancer frequency) to be realized.

11.1.2. Cancer of the Breast, Corpus Uteri and Prostate

Etiopathogenesis of these neoplasms seems to be even more complex. Hormonal, host factors are probably paramount in the development of these cancers. Both the production of hormones and the status of the organs on which these hormones act and, in consequence, the response of those organs to the hormones, are, however, dependent to a large extent on environmental factors, especially on nutrition. It seems that a diet rich in animal proteins and fats favors the development of these cancers or, in the case of prostate cancer, promotes the transformation of asymptomatic, latent, lowly malignant forms into symptomatic, more malignant ones. Such an hypothesis is further supported by the positive correlation between these cancers and cancer of the colon and rectum, in the development of which nutrition also seems to be an important factor.

The hypothesis that these cancers are associated with nutrition and dietary habits may account for the low but increasing frequency of their occurrence in Poland, especially in rural areas, as well as for the increase observed in Polish migrants.

11.1.3 Cancer of the Uterine Cervix

Genesis of this disease seems to depend on a factor transmitted by coitus, but it is not yet clear whether childbearing also increases the risk of this cancer. As discussed in Chapter 9.6, the hypothesis of viral infection is consistent with epidemiologic observations. Data currently available, however, do not permit identification of this postulated infectious factor, nor do they enable us to check whether the viral hypothesis can account for the high risk of this cancer prevailing in Poland or its decrease in Polish migrants.

11.1.4. Lung Cancer

It may be assumed that a large majority of the cases of this cancer in Poland is related to cigarette smoking. Because of its rapid increase in frequency, lung cancer is presently overtaking other cancers in males; and the continued rapid increase in cigarette consumption indicates that this increase in frequency will continue in both males and females. Prevention of lung cancer through a decrease in cigarette consumption is not easy to achieve, but was recently verified in practice: a decrease of cigarette consumption among British physicians was followed by a decrease in lung cancer mortality [40].

Although occupational factors and air pollution currently play only a secondary part, in comparison with tobacco smoking, they seem to increase lung cancer risk more for smokers than for nonsmokers.

11.2. Rationale for the Continued Study of Cancer Epidemiology in Poland

The results of epidemiologic investigations of cancer obtained thus far have demonstrated their value in the campaign against cancer. Such investigations have already led to the identification of a number of carcinogenic factors. In turn, the elimination of these factors or limitation of exposure to them has permitted the successful cancer prevention in some instances. Some examples include the relation between carcinogenic hydrocarbons and skin and lung cancer; between aniline dyes and urinary bladder cancer; between ionizing radiation and radioactive substances and cancer of the skin, lung, and thyroid as well as leukemia and sarcomas; between tobacco smoking and lung cancer.

Carcinogenic factors discovered to date account for only a small part of cancer incidence, especially if we leave out discoveries about tobacco smoking. The results of epidemiologic studies, including the present study, are, nevertheless, significant, having shown, among other things, the primary importance of environmental factors in cancer etiopathogenesis. Because of epidemiologic studies, we can now estimate that approximately 80 percent of all malignant tumors are likely to be conditioned environmentally and, in theory, preventable [74,75]. Previous experience suggests that further epidemiologic studies will lead to the discovery of these environmental factors, and permit the introduction of preventive measures leading to a substantial decrease in the frequency of cancer occurrence.

Expected ecologic and demographic changes also demonstrate the need to continue and expand the study of cancer epidemiology. Given the present ecologic and demographic conditions, the development of such studies is justified, but these conditions are by no means static; their dynamism is a characteristic feature of our time. Previous experience indicates that changes in our environment, caused by increasing industrialization or altered habits and customs, are often connected with an increased exposure to carcinogenic factors. They can be either occupational factors, affecting only small groups of persons who come in contact with them, or factors affecting large population groups — like water and air pollution or danger from chemical additives to food or spread of some harmful habits. Detecting the increase in cancer risk early and establishing its causes requires thorough epidemiologic studies and surveillance.

In addition, the demographic situation in Poland demonstrates the need for a more intensive campaign against cancer.

Cancer caused nearly 44,000 deaths in Poland in 1969 and 47,000 in 1971. The estimated number of new cases was over 60,000 in 1969 [98,99]. A substantial increase in these numbers can be expected, even in the absence of an increase in exposure to carcinogenic factors, because the number of persons over 60 in Poland has doubled in the last two decades and, cancer being a disease of older people in particular, its social importance increases as the proportion of old persons in the population rises. A further increase in the proportion of older people is expected and will result in a substantial increase in cancer incidence and mortality, further increasing the social importance of this disease.

The need for a more intensive fight against cancer cannot be questioned. It should be obvious, even if the proposition is not so generally accepted, that cancer prevention, based on detection and elimination of carcinogenic factors, is as important in the fight against cancer, as earlier detection or improved methods of treatment. Because their aim is to find new methods of cancer prevention, studies of cancer epidemiology should be carried forward.

Continuing study of the epidemiology of all the cancers discussed in this book seems warranted in Poland. The high risk of stomach cancer and of uterine cervix cancer observed in Poland requires explanation. These two cancers, together with lung cancer are the most common cancers in Poland. Studies of their epidemiology will not only be both timely and socially important, they will also be more easily facilitated by the availability of large amounts of data.

The increase in the frequency of occurrence of cancers of the intestinal tract, breast or prostate indicates that these, together with the lungs, will soon be the most frequent primary cancer sites in Poland. These cancers should also have priority in the planning of epidemiologic studies.

The epidemiology of lung cancer is understood well enough to show how most cases of this disease could be prevented. There are justifiable fears, however, that growing industrialization and its related environmental changes may lead to an increase in lung cancer risk among some occupational groups or in some geographic regions. Lung cancer should not be neglected in future epidemiologic studies.

Poland offers particularly good opportunities for studies of cancer epidemiology because of special features such as:

1. When compared with cancer risk in other countries, risk in Poland is unusually high for some cancer sites, such as the stomach or cervix uteri and low for others such as the intestines, breast, and prostate. The explanation of these differences in cancer risk may provide more information about the etiopathogenesis of these cancers and identify the carcinogenic factors.

2. Changes in cancer risks are particularly great in Poland, providing an advantageous setting for epidemiologic research.

3. Industrial development and social and environmental change in Poland do not always follow the patterns established in other countries. This situation may help to demonstrate the significance in cancer etiopathogenesis of suspected factors, many of which may appear or disappear in Poland at different times than in the other countries.

4. Population redistribution within Poland, besides the migration from rural to urban areas observed in most countries, was characterized by large movements of population during and after the Second World War. These movements, generally from east to west, were in some respects comparable to the east to west movements of the pioneers in the United States but took place in a much shorter time. This population redistribution offers additional possibilities for studies of cancer risk displacements related to migration.

5. Polish migrants are one of the largest groups of foreign-born migrants in the United States, and sizable groups are also to be found in other countries including Brasil, Canada, Argentina, France and Great Britain [182]. The existence of these groups creates the possibility for comparative studies of the shifts in cancer risk connected with migration to different environments.

11.3. General Conclusions about Future Studies

Some general conclusions about future studies of cancer epidemiology and etiopathogenesis can be drawn from the preceding chapters.

Studies of cancer occurrence require a more specific classification of tumors than one listing only the organ of primary site, because various types of cancer can develop in one organ, differing not only in primary localization, morphology and prognosis, but also in their epidemiologic characteristics [16,32]. Such differences are concealed if these various cancer types cannot be considered separately. Epidemiologic studies therefore require classifications by tumor localization within the organ (in which part of the stomach or segment of the colon), morphology (diffuse versus intestinal type stomach cancer), clinical characteristics (symptomatic or asymptomatic prostate cancer). At the same time, the morphologic criteria which permit the identification of cancer types such as pre- and postmenopausal breast cancer which differ in epidemiologic characteristics should be sought for.

Information on the morphology of the tumor-free parts of an organ in which cancer developed may be helpful in the identification of morphologic lesions favoring or accompanying cancer development. For such studies, the preservation of entire organs is useful, because it permits later examination for additional information which initially might not have been of interest in the course of the study.

Identification of high- and low-risk populations with respect to some cancer can be helpful in the detection of carcinogenic factors, while an increase in cancer risk for a given population (such as workers at a specific occupation group or residents of a particular area), if noticed, is an alarm signaling a change in the epidemiologic situation which calls for rapid action.

Detailed information on cancer localization and morphology, as well as on its occurrence in various populations, is easier to obtain from cancer registries than from mortality statistics. These two sources of information, however, are complementary. Mortality statistics present a better picture of cancer distribution throughout the country, but cancer registration offers more detailed and reliable data for the selected regions of Poland. Cancer registration also permits the evaluation of treatment results in a defined population; such studies have recently been initiated in Poland [96].

The consistency of results, based on available mortality statistics in Poland and on cancer registration in the selected regions of the country, was demonstrated in the previous chapters. The detailed and up-to-date demographic data of the 1970 census will allow computation of the age-specific incidence and mortality rates not only by districts but also by counties, even for the old age groups, permitting still more precise comparisons of the mortality and incidence statistics.

Utilisation of mortality statistics in epidemiologic investigations, on other diseases as well as cancer, would be much improved if the degree of accuracy and reliability of death certification with respect to age, sex and residence of the deceased were determined and if it were also known to what extent available diagnostic information was utilized for death certification.

The frequency with which morphologic lesions preceding the appearance of symptomatic cancer occur in a healthy population may be used as a measure of cancer risk in that population. Such lesions may include latent, asymptomatic cancer, precancerous lesions, or merely the effects of the action of identified or unidentified carcinogenic factors, or factors associated with them that may not lead to cancerization at all. Examples of such lesions include intestinal metaplasia of the stomach mucosa, intestinal polyps, or yellow coloration of finger tips, although, of course, cigarette smokers are better identified by a few questions then by inspection of their hands.

Morphologic lesions preceding the appearance of symptomatic cancer and signaling its increased risk are present not only earlier but also more frequently than cancer; these two factors facilitate the search for conditions favoring their appearance.

The frequency of occurrence of other host characteristics associated with a particular cancer, favoring or only preceding cancer appearance, may be utilized as another measure of the risk of this cancer in a population. Studies of steroid excretion, directed to measuring breast cancer risk, may be cited as an example. Better knowledge of such characteristics, hormonal, immunologic, chromosomal and the like, may increase our understanding of cancer etiopathogenesis. Furthermore, the identification of such host characteristics may help to identify persons having an increased cancer risk and to offer them either preventive measures or a careful follow up to ensure early detection and treatment.

Even detailed knowledge both of the occurrence of a particular cancer and of the morphologic lesions preceding it is not enough to determine its etiopathogenesis. For that purpose, comparative studies designed to identify carcinogenic factors are required. They may consist of comparison of the occurrence of both the factor and cancer under study in various populations or time periods, or of case-control and cohort studies (see Chapter 1.2). In conducting such studies, it seems advantageous to include detailed morphologic data concerning type of cancer, co-existing lesions in the same organ and in other organs as well as laboratory measurements of such factors as hormonal and immunologic status. The utilization of data linkage techniques [2] would also be advantagous, permitting the study of cancer occurrence in persons with specific characteristics of interest such as history of hospitalization for tuberculosis or of treatment with isoniazid.

Difficulties connected with identifying carcinogenic factors and interpreting the results of such comparative studies suggest the advisability of utilizing situations favorable to epidemiologic investigations. An example of one such situation is the similarity of cancer occurrence in Poland and Japan repeatedly mentioned throughout the present study. This similarity is surprising in view of great differences between the two countries in so many respects, and this situation indicates that cooperative Polish-Japanese studies of cancer epidemiology might be fruitful.

Higginson [73] has pointed out the difficulties inherent in discovering associations between cancer and those factors which are pervasive in the population studied. For example, demonstration of the association between smoking and lung cancer would be difficult if all adults were smokers. Analogous situations may be one of the reasons for the poor results of studies of the association between dietary habits and cancer of the stomach or intestinal tract. Such difficulties may not be so great in populations in which the risk of the cancer under study is changing, indicating a change in the prevalence of the factors which affect chances of the development of this cancer.

Difficulties related to the prevalence of a specific carcinogenic factor can also be partly circumvented through comparative studies of migrants between countries with different levels of cancer risk, and also presumably in the prevalence of the factors bearing on that risk.

Migrant population studies facilitate the determination and disentanglement of the effects of varied environmental changes on cancer risk. Such studies require the knowledge of cancer occurrence in both the country of birth and the host country. Registration of cancer incidence in the selected regions of Poland can furnish more detailed data on primary location, histology, and even on prognosis, than is available from mortality statistics. Similar data on cancer incidence in Polish migrants living in some areas of the United States are expected to be available within the next few years, permitting a better evaluation of migration related changes in cancer risk. Investigation of the effects of internal migration in Poland will also soon be possible because information on place of birth was included in the 1970 census.

The next step should be the special comparative studies, already mentioned, designed to determine the prevalence of lesions and host characteristics preceding cancer appearance and of suspected carcinogenic factors, comparing these prevalences among migrants and in their country of birth and of adoption.

A factor that should be included in studies of migrant populations is age at migration, which permits estimation of the length of exposure of the migrant to both his old and new environments. If possible, the second generation of Polish migrants to the United States should also be included in the studies, and the investigations should also be broadened to cover other countries with large Polish populations.

Laboratory studies and animal experiments designed to identify carcinogens and to elucidate cancer etiopathogenesis may well supplement the epidemiologic studies discussed above. Some examples, related to stomach cancer, might be chemical and biological studies of suspected foods and experimental studies of the effects of dietary deficiencies and the mechanisms of their possible carcinogenic action.

Epidemiologic observations may inspire the creation of experimental models such as experiments with animals to verify the hypothesis that vitamin A deficiencies are instrumental in the development of some cancers [146,148]. Comparative studies of the epidemiology of cancer in man and animals, such as a study of breast cancer in men and in dogs, have also developed recently [155].

Appropriate linking of epidemiologic, laboratory, and animal experimental studies should greatly increase our knowledge of human cancer etiopathogenesis. Without such a linking the value of experimental and laboratory investigations is restricted, for it is well known that the results of studies on one species cannot be transfered to other, even allied, species. Furthermore, man lives under quite different conditions from those under which such experiments are conducted. The results of experiments on pure genetical strains, for example, suggest a much higher significance of genetic factors in cancer etiopathogenesis than it is apparent from observations of cancer in man.

Another problem has been commented upon by Kotin [101]: "the demonstration of a carcinogen in the environment need not inevitably connote a biological effect". The effectiveness of a chemical carcinogen may depend on the simultaneous operation of other factors, and also on its "biological availability — the ability to gain host entry, reach target organs, and interact with cellular components concerned with malignant transformation" in a suitable form and effective physico-chemical condition, all of which may be determined, among others, by the size of the particles, their solubility, and chemical reactions inside and outside the organism.

In general it may be concluded that it is dangerous to infer human cancer etiopathogenesis only from the results of experimental and laboratory studies without supporting observations on cancer occurrence in man.

For the purpose of presenting directions proposed for future research, epidemiologic observations suggest a particular grouping of the cancers discussed.

The rationale for studying stomach and intestinal tract cancer jointly is indicated both by their contrasting epidemiologic features and by their probable association with dietary habits and nutrition. Future investigations should be primarily directed to elucidate what dietary changes preceded the changes in risk of these cancers. This may be made easier by the fact that these changes, usually the results of improving socioeconomic conditions, involved many diet components indeed, but usually not all at the same time and to the same degree. Other questions requiring answers include the following:

1. Does our diet contain carcinogens? It seems that in Poland laboratory and animal experimental studies should give priority to potatoes and pickled foods.

2. Do dietary deficiences favor the development of stomach cancer? If so, which ones?

3. How do changes in dietary habits from the old ones, connected with a low risk of intestinal tract cancer, to the new ones, associated with its increasing risk, influence peristalsis, and the chemical composition and bacteria of intestinal contents?

Similarities in epidemiologic features between cancers of breast, uterine corpus, and prostate indicate that their etiopathogenesis may also be similar, and suggest the advisability of studying them jointly. It seems that here, too, dietary habits and nutrition require much attention. Future studies should cover, among others, the following questions:

1. What possible dietary components influence development of these tumors?

2. What part do other factors play in the etiopathogenesis of these cancers? For instance, why does childbearing decrease the risk of breast and uterine corpus cancer?

3. How do dietary habits, and other factors bearing on the risk of these cancers, effect human hormonal state?

4. What is the relation of the effect of these factors to the age at which they act?

Future epidemiologic studies on uterine cervix cancer should be concerned primarily with the search for the infectious agent which is the probable cause of this cancer. Combined epidemiologic, virusologic and possibly hormonal studies seem advisable.

Lung cancer presents a different problem, because its etiopathogenesis is known to an extent sufficient to propose steps which could prevent most cases of this cancer. Nevertheless, studies on the association between lung cancer and smoking are still continuing, because lung cancer in smokers is presently the best source of information on human cancer etiopathogenesis and is often defined as a natural experiment — not always well planned and conducted, but covering a very large body of material. This makes it possible to estimate the dependence of cancer risk on such variables as intensity of the carcinogen action, duration of this action, even cessation of exposure in those who stopped smoking — the dependence of the risk on each of these variables and on their combinations.

For future studies of lung cancer epidemiology in Poland, two avenues of approach seem to be most promising:

1. Utilisation of the effects of the singular population redistributions in an attempt to elucidate the "migration effect", discussed on page 91.

2. Follow-up of the occurrence of lung cancer and of lesions preceding its appearance, in order to detect as early as possible the eventual increase in lung cancer risk, which may follow industrialization and rapid environmental changes.

11.4. Final Conclusions

1. In comparison with other countries, Poland is characterized by a low, but increasing risk of cancer of the intestinal tract, breast, corpus uteri, and prostate. The risk of cancer of the stomach and of the uterine cervix in Poland is high; only in recent years has stomach cancer risk shown some decline. The increase in lung cancer risk is similar in Poland to that observed in other countries.

2. Among Polish migrants to the United States and to Australia, to countries with a different pattern of cancer risks, site-specific displacements of risks are observed. Stomach cancer mortality among Polish-born Americans in 1950 was as high as in Poland; ten years later it had decreased, but continued to be more closely aligned to the high rates in Poland than to the low rates prevailing for the natives of the host country. The intestinal tract cancer mortality of these migrants has risen to equal the much higher risk prevailing for United States natives. Mortality from cancer of the breast, uterine corpus and prostate among these Polish migrants to the United States has also increased from the low level reported for Poland, but has not yet reached the high level characteristic of United States natives. On the other hand, lung cancer mortality among Polish-born Americans was higher than either in Poland or among native Americans, especially in the older age groups.

Displacements in cancer mortality noted among Polish migrants to Australia were similar to those for Polish-born Americans.

3. Geographical differences and changes over time in cancer occurrence, exemplified by the data presented for Poland and Polish migrants, point to the primary importance of environmental factors in their etiopathogenesis. Knowledge of these factors, however, is still fragmentary. Dietary habits and nutrition seem to play an important and similar part in the etiopathogenesis of cancer of the intestinal tract, breast, uterine corpus, and prostate; for stomach cancer they are also probably as important, but the mechanism of their action is likely to be quite different. Uterine cervix cancer seems to depend on infectious, possibly viral, factors. The association between lung cancer and cigarette smoking is known quite well.

4. Both the results of the earlier epidemiologic studies and expected environmental and demographic changes demonstrate the necessity of continuing and expanding the study of the epidemiology of these cancers in Poland. The great differences between the frequency and time trends of the occurrence of these cancers in Poland and in other countries, the singular population redistributions connected with the Second World War, and, last but not least, the sizable Polish migrant groups in countries with varied environments, create especially favorable conditions for such studies in Poland and among Polish migrants.

5. Future studies should link the epidemiologic, pathomorphologic, environmental, laboratory, and animal experimental investigations more closely than they have in the past. Such complex studies, carried out simultaneously in various populations and environments, should lead to a much more rapid identification of carcinogenic factors, and permit successful cancer prevention.

Appendix

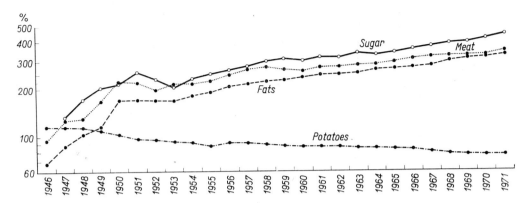

Fig. A-1. Average annual consumption per capita of potatoes, meat, fats and sugar, in Poland, expressed as a percentage of consumption in 1938 [140].

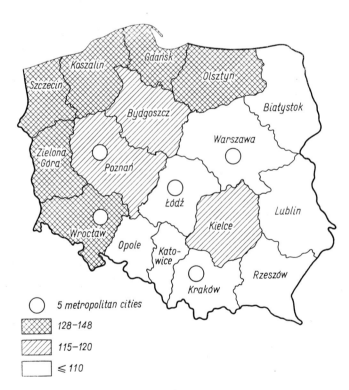

Fig. A-2. Age-adjusted fertility rates per 1000 women aged 15-49, by district of residence in 1950–51 in Poland. Standard: age distribution of 15–49 year-old women of the whole country at the same time [184].

Table A-1

Population in thousands of Poland from the Censuses on December 6, 1960, and on December 8, 1970 by sex, residence, and age [18,129].

A. Census of 1960

Age	Total		Males			Females		
	Thousand	Percent	Total	Urban	Rural	Total	Urban	Rural
Total	29,405.7	100.0	14,058.6	6,735.0	7,323.6	15,347.2	7,471.1	7,876.1
0–4	3,381.1	11.5	1,728.9	764.2	964.7	1,652.1	727.3	924.9
5–9	3,514.7	12.0	1,792.7	822.7	970.0	1,722,0	788.8	933.2
10–14	3,040.0	10.3	1,547.0	696.9	850.1	1,493.0	677.2	815.7
15–19	1,924.7	6.5	968.2	503.7	464.5	956.5	485.6	470.9
20–24	1,950.7	6.6	862.8	454.5	408.3	1,087.9	568.7	519.2
25–29	2,282.2	7.8	1,133.5	611.4	522.1	1,148.6	622.2	526.4
30–34	2,310.5	7.9	1,122.8	608.6	514.2	1,187.7	632.6	555.1
35–39	2,054.2	7.0	949.1	502.4	446.7	1,105.0	576.4	528.7
40–44	1,349.7	4.6	624.5	303.5	321.0	725.1	357.1	368.0
45–49	1,621.3	5.5	743.6	354.0	389.6	877.6	427.6	450.1
50–54	1,696.6	5.8	796.7	358.9	437.8	899.9	431.1	468.9
55–59	1,413.7	4.8	648.0	282.1	365.9	765.7	361.5	404.2
60–64	1,093.9	3.7	466.5	194.8	271.7	627.4	295.4	332.0
65–69	730.8	2.5	295.5	122.1	173.4	435.3	208.6	226.7
70–74	513.6	1.8	194.0	80.3	113.6	319.6	151.5	168.1
75–79	292.2	1.0	105.0	43.3	61.8	187.2	88.5	98.7
80–84	141.7	0.5	47.7	19.4	28.3	94.0	44.4	49.5
85+	71.3	0.2	21.1	8.2	12.9	50.2	22.3	27.9
Age unknown	23.0	0.1	10.8	3.9	6.9	12.2	4.2	8.0

B. Census of 1970

Age	Total		Males			Females		
Total	32,642.3	100.0	15.853.6	8,172.3	7,681.4	16,788.7	8,892.3	7,896.3
0–4	2,505.6	7.7	1,280.5	583.1	697.4	1,225.1	555.1	670.0
5–9	2,732.7	8.4	1,398.5	637.8	760.7	1,334.2	609.5	724.7
10–14	3,389.1	10.4	1,730.1	822.1	908.0	1,659.0	787.3	871.7
15–19	3,477.2	10.7	1,771.6	995.6	776.0	1,705.6	979.8	725.8
20–24	2,957.4	9.1	1,498.8	825.3	673.5	1,458.6	849.5	609.0
25–29	1,888.2	5.8	948.8	548.1	400.7	939.4	566.6	372.8
30–34	2,155.1	6.6	1,076.0	618.8	457.1	1,079.1	641.0	438.1
35–39	2,256.6	6.9	1,127.0	644.8	482.2	1,129.6	651.0	478.6
40–44	2,255.8	6.9	1,097.4	612.5	484.9	1,158.4	639.2	519.2
45–49	1,986.0	6.1	914.8	492.5	422.3	1,071.2	574.4	496.8
50–54	1,281.0	3.9	587.4	289.2	298.2	693.6	351.4	342.2
55–59	1,501.2	4.6	674.1	324.6	349.5	827.1	419.4	407.7
60–64	1,499.8	4.6	676.3	308.5	367.8	823.5	415.1	408.4
65–69	1,163.2	3.6	498.2	221.1	277.1	665.0	333.0	331.9
70–74	796.6	2.4	306.5	131.6	174.9	490.1	247.0	243.1
75–79	441.2	1.4	155.0	66.6	88.4	286.2	147.7	138.5
80–84	227.9	0.7	72.5	31.8	40.7	155.4	80.2	75.2
85+	106.8	0.4	29.9	13.3	16.6	76.9	39.5	37.4
Age unknown	20.7	0.0	10.2	4.9	5.3	10.5	5.5	5.0

Table A-2

Population of the areas covered by the Polish regional cancer registries, by sex and age, on December 31, 1965[89, 90, 95, 206]

Age (years)	Region							
	Warszawa City		Katowice District		Kraków District		4 Rural Areas	
	males	females	males	females	males	females	males	females
Total	580,700	671,900	1673,700	1727,600	1186,700	1271,700	257,548	277,860
0–4	34,900	32,500	139,200	130,600	114,800	108,600	27,003	25,561
5–9	52,300	49,400	168,200	157,500	129,400	124,300	29,240	28,128
10–14	60,700	58,100	164,300	157,100	130,500	125,900	30,067	29,197
15–19	50,900	50,300	138,100	132,500	112,300	108,400	26,321	25,910
20–24	35,000	41,500	132,800	118,400	78,600	77,800	18,157	18,531
25–29	47,200	50,400	169,300	132,400	88,500	87,200	16,783	17,600
30–34	51,200	54,900	148,200	127,800	89,300	91,000	17,276	18,002
35–39	58,100	57,800	130,300	125,800	85,600	90,200	17,093	17,935
40–44	45,800	50,400	97,100	120,100	72,900	83,600	14,441	17,559
45–49	26,000	33,100	62,300	79,400	46,000	55,200	9,568	11,969
50–54	30,400	41,200	79,600	103,000	57,900	70,000	12,083	14,664
55–59	32,700	43,900	83,200	102,600	61,700	71,900	12,708	15,108
60–64	55,500	108,400	67,400	85,700	50,700	63,800	10,821	13,161
65–69			45,200	65,500	34,400	50,000	7,674	10,368
70+			48,500	89,200	34,100	63,800	8,313	14,167

Table A-3

Warszawa City. Average annual incidence per 100,000 by age, sex and primary cancer localization, 1965–66[94]

ICD, 1955 rev.	Site	All ages	0–	5–	10–	15–	20–	25–	30–	35–	40–	45–	50–	55–	60+
							M A L E S								
140–205	All sites whereof:	205.2	15.8	10.5	10.7	14.7	18.6	24.4	30.3	55.1	112.4	201.9	282.9	501.5	1343.2
151	stomach	35.5	0.0	0.0	0.0	0.0	0.0	3.2	2.0	5.2	13.1	30.8	46.1	79.5	262.2
152,153	intestines	6.6	0.0	0.0	0.0	0.0	1.4	0.0	3.9	0.9	3.3	17.3	8.2	18.3	37.8
154	rectum	5.5	0.0	0.0	0.0	0.0	1.4	1.1	0.0	1.7	2.2	3.8	14.8	13.8	34.2
162,163	lung	44.9	0.0	0.0	0.8	0.0	0.0	0.0	0.0	7.7	25.1	34.6	51.0	136.1	315.3
177	prostate	11.3	0.0	1.9	0.0	0.0	0.0	0.0	0.0	0.0	0.0	1.9	4.9	4.6	109.9
Rate per case			1.43	0.96	0.82	0.98	1.43	1.06	0.98	0.86	1.09	1.92	1.64	1.53	0.90
							F E M A L E S								
140–205	All sites whereof:	274.7	20.0	7.1	12.9	13.9	24.1	53.6	90.2	136.7	253.0	302.1	394.4	478.4	970.5
151	stomach	25.7	1.5	0.0	0.0	1.0	0.0	2.0	2.7	3.5	5.0	7.6	9.7	29.6	134.2
152,153	intestines	10.7	0.0	0.0	0.0	0.0	0.0	0.0	0.0	3.5	4.0	3.0	7.3	15.9	52.6
154	rectum	5.6	0.0	0.0	0.0	0.0	2.4	0.0	0.0	2.6	6.0	3.0	9.7	9.1	21.2
162,163	lung	11.9	0.0	0.0	0.0	0.0	0.0	0.0	0.9	3.5	6.9	6.0	18.2	17.1	52.6
170	breast	37.6	0.0	0.0	0.0	1.0	1.2	1.0	8.2	18.2	55.6	69.5	85.0	86.6	102.4
171	cervix uteri	48.2	0.0	0.0	0.0	0.0	6.0	32.7	55.6	77.0	102.2	98.2	92.2	82.0	66.0
172	corpus uteri	9.6	0.0	0.0	0.0	0.0	0.0	0.0	0.0	0.0	6.0	12.1	25.5	22.8	33.7
173–174	uterus-other and unspecified	4.3	0.0	0.0	0.0	0.0	0.0	0.0	0.9	0.0	2.0	6.0	7.3	5.7	18.5
Rate per case			1.54	1.01	0.86	0.99	1.20	0.99	0.91	0.87	0.99	1.51	1.21	1.14	0.46

Table A-4

Katowice District. Average annual incidence per 100,000 by age, sex and primary cancer localization, 1965–66[206]

ICD 1955 rev.	Site	All ages	0–	1–	5–	10–	15–	20–	25–	30–	35–	40–	45–	50–	55–	60–	65–	70+
								MALES										
140–205	All sites	126.5	13.0	11.1	8.9	5.2	9.4	9.8	15.4	33.7	44.1	95.8	182.2	313.4	414.7	635.8	691.4	758.8
	whereof:																	
151	stomach	28.2	0.0	0.9	0.0	0.0	0.0	0.0	0.9	7.1	6.1	17.5	39.3	79.8	95.6	154.3	149.3	188.7
152, 153	intestines	4.5	0.0	0.0	0.0	0.3	0.4	1.1	0.9	0.7	1.2	2.6	3.2	11.3	15.6	25.9	16.6	34.0
154	rectum	5.3	0.0	0.0	0.0	0.0	0.0	0.0	0.6	1.0	1.5	3.1	4.8	10.1	11.4	31.9	36.5	47.4
162, 163	lung	27.5	1.9	0.0	0.3	0.0	0.0	0.0	0.6	2.0	7.3	20.6	50.6	69.7	105.2	160.2	186.9	115.5
177	prostate	3.9	0.0	0.0	0.3	0.0	0.0	0.0	0.0	0.0	0.0	0.5	0.0	1.9	9.0	15.6	32.1	61.9
Rate per case			1.86	0.45	0.30	0.30	0.36	0.38	0.30	0.34	0.38	0.51	0.80	0.63	0.60	0.74	1.11	1.03
								FEMALES										
140–205	All sites	145.8	9.9	5.7	7.9	6.7	7.2	17.3	34.4	62.6	118.0	176.9	222.9	295.1	361.6	419.5	511.5	466.9
	whereof:																	
151	stomach	17.5	0.0	0.0	0.0	0.0	0.0	0.0	1.1	2.3	6.8	10.8	18.9	26.7	34.1	61.3	93.1	94.7
152, 153	intestines	4.4	0.0	0.0	0.0	0.0	0.0	0.0	0.4	0.4	0.8	3.7	6.3	7.3	14.1	18.1	13.7	20.2
154	rectum	4.8	0.0	0.0	0.3	0.0	0.4	0.8	0.4	0.4	1.2	3.3	4.4	9.2	14.1	15.8	20.6	21.3
162, 163	lung	3.4	0.0	0.0	0.0	0.0	0.4	0.8	0.4	0.4	2.8	4.6	2.5	3.4	8.3	8.8	16.8	15.1
170	breast	19.8	0.0	0.0	0.0	0.0	0.0	1.3	1.1	10.6	15.1	35.4	52.9	49.5	56.0	55.4	44.3	40.4
171	cervix uteri	34.9	0.0	0.0	0.0	0.3	0.0	3.4	18.9	32.5	62.4	74.5	83.8	85.9	75.5	64.2	64.1	37.6
172	corpus uteri	5.6	0.0	0.0	0.0	0.0	0.0	0.0	0.0	0.0	1.6	1.7	3.8	13.1	25.3	27.4	28.2	9.0
173–174	uterus-other and unspecified	3.0	0.0	0.0	0.0	0.0	0.0	0.0	0.0	0.4	1.6	3.3	6.3	8.7	6.8	7.6	12.2	10.7
Rate per case			1.98	0.47	0.32	0.32	0.38	0.42	0.38	0.39	0.40	0.42	0.63	0.49	0.49	0.58	0.76	0.56

Table A-5
Kraków City and District. Average annual incidence per 100,000 by age, sex and primary cancer localization, 1965-66[89]

ICD, 1955 rev.	Site	All ages	0-	1-	5-	10-	15-	20-	25-	30-	35-	40-	45-	50-	55-	60-	65-	70+
								MALES										
140–205	All sites whereof:	149.2	2.2	18.0	13.5	5.7	13.8	17.2	20.9	29.7	59.6	113.9	206.5	321.2	512.2	668.6	893.9	788.9
151	Stomach	33.7	0.0	0.0	0.0	0.0	0.4	0.6	0.6	5.0	11.1	19.9	42.4	76.9	139.4	169.6	229.7	152.5
152, 153	intestines	4.9	0.0	0.0	0.0	0.0	0.0	0.0	0.0	0.6	1.8	6.2	3.3	11.3	16.3	22.6	33.4	29.4
154	rectum	3.2	0.0	0.0	0.0	0.0	0.0	0.0	0.0	0.6	1.8	0.7	2.2	6.0	13.8	10.8	21.8	27.9
162, 163	lung	27.6	0.0	0.0	0.0	0.0	0.0	0.0	0.0	1.7	7.0	16.5	34.8	63.9	110.2	159.8	193.3	111.4
177	prostate	4.2	0.0	0.0	0.0	0.0	0.0	0.0	0.0	0.0	0.0	0.0	0.0	0.9	6.5	15.8	37.8	71.8
Rate per case			2.18	0.54	0.39	0.38	0.45	0.64	0.56	0.56	0.58	0.69	1.09	0.86	0.81	0.99	1.45	1.47
									FEMALES									
140–205	All sites whereof:	141.2	2.3	12.1	4.4	6.0	10.6	10.3	26.4	54.9	100.9	174.6	253.6	307.9	358.1	433.4	509.0	467.9
151	stomach	16.9	0.0	0.0	0.0	0.0	0.0	0.0	0.0	2.7	11.1	14.4	25.4	27.9	49.4	61.9	74.0	71.3
152, 153	intestines	4.3	0.0	0.0	0.0	0.0	0.0	0.0	0.6	0.5	1.1	1.8	5.4	6.4	12.5	12.5	22.0	25.9
154	rectum	3.3	0.0	0.0	0.0	0.0	0.0	0.0	0.0	0.5	0.6	3.6	7.2	10.7	9.0	12.5	9.0	11.8
162, 163	lung	4.6	0.0	0.0	0.0	0.0	0.5	0.0	0.6	0.0	0.6	3.6	7.2	9.3	11.1	16.5	21.0	24.3
170	breast	21.5	0.0	0.0	0.0	0.4	0.0	0.0	1.7	9.3	15.0	40.7	50.7	54.3	60.5	62.7	60.0	55.6
171	cervix uteri	23.5	0.0	0.0	0.0	0.0	0.0	1.9	6.9	17.6	34.4	59.2	61.6	57.9	60.5	54.1	58.0	20.4
172	corpus uteri	5.5	0.0	0.0	0.0	0.0	0.0	0.0	0.6	0.0	0.6	3.0	9.1	19.3	23.6	22.7	18.0	11.0
173–174	uterus-other and unspecified	1.4	0.0	0.0	0.0	0.0	0.0	0.0	0.6	0.5	2.2	0.6	2.7	2.1	7.0	3.9	3.0	3.1
Rate per case			2.33	0.57	0.40	0.40	0.46	0.64	0.57	0.55	0.55	0.60	0.91	0.71	0.70	0.78	1.00	0.78

Table A-6
Four Rural Areas.
Average annual incidence per 100,000 by age, sex and primary cancer localization, 1965-66[90]

ICD, 1955 rev.	Site	All ages	0-	5-	10-	15-	20-	25-	30-	35-	40-	45-	50-	55-	60-	65-	70+
									M A L E S								
140–205	All sites whereof:	157.1	18.5	10.3	6.7	9.5	19.3	17.9	43.4	49.7	110.8	172.4	277.2	499.7	628.4	990.4	1154.8
151	stomach	45.4	0.0	0.0	0.0	0.0	2.8	0.0	2.9	11.7	17.3	67.9	78.6	181.0	249.5	306.2	264.6
152, 153	intestines	2.9	0.0	0.0	0.0	0.0	2.8	3.0	0.0	0.0	0.0	0.0	4.1	7.9	4.6	26.1	30.1
154	rectum	3.1	0.0	0.0	0.0	0.0	0.0	3.0	0.0	0.0	0.0	0.0	0.0	11.8	9.2	13.0	48.1
162, 163	lung	25.0	0.0	0.0	0.0	0.0	0.0	0.0	2.9	0.0	13.8	36.6	62.1	114.1	97.0	156.4	168.4
177	prostate	8.2	0.0	0.0	0.0	0.0	0.0	0.0	0.0	0.0	3.5	0.0	4.1	3.9	37.0	71.7	120.3
	Rate per case		1.85	1.71	1.66	1.90	2.75	2.98	2.89	2.93	3.46	5.23	4.14	3.93	4.62	6.52	6.01
									F E M A L E S								
140–205	All sites whereof:	149.2	11.7	3.6	3.4	11.6	10.8	31.2	58.3	83.6	202.2	200.5	259.1	370.7	550.9	631.8	578.8
151	stomach	25.2	0.0	0.0	0.0	0.0	0.0	0.0	2.8	11.2	19.9	29.2	20.5	76.1	121.6	101.3	137.6
152, 153	intestines	4.0	0.0	0.0	0.0	0.0	0.0	0.0	0.0	0.0	5.7	4.2	3.4	6.6	11.4	28.9	24.7
154	rectum	3.6	0.0	0.0	0.0	0.0	0.0	0.0	0.0	0.0	0.0	0.0	0.0	9.9	11.4	24.1	31.8
162, 163	lung	4.5	0.0	0.0	0.0	0.0	0.0	0.0	2.8	11.2	0.0	4.2	10.2	16.5	11.4	38.6	14.1
170	breast	16.9	0.0	0.0	0.0	0.0	0.0	8.5	11.1	11.2	31.3	50.1	44.3	62.9	45.6	57.9	24.7
171	cervix uteri	20.9	0.0	0.0	0.0	0.0	0.0	0.0	16.7	41.8	57.0	37.6	61.4	39.7	68.4	38.6	24.7
172	corpus uteri	7.2	0.0	0.0	0.0	0.0	0.0	0.0	2.8	0.0	5.7	0.0	30.7	29.8	34.2	24.1	17.6
173, 174	Uterus-other and unspecified	3.4	0.0	0.0	0.0	0.0	0.0	2.8	0.0	0.0	2.8	4.2	0.0	16.5	7.6	28.9	10.6
	Rate per case		1.96	1.78	1.71	1.93	2.70	2.84	2.78	2.79	2.85	4.18	3.41	3.31	3.80	4.82	3.53

Table A-7
Poland (total country), 1967-69.
Average annual mortality per 100,000 by age, sex and primary cancer localization

Age columns span 0-4 through 85+.

ICD 1955 rev.	Site	Total	0-4	5-9	10-14	15-19	20-24	25-29	30-34	35-39	40-44	45-49	50-54	55-59	60-64	65-69	70-74	75-79	80-84	85+
								MALES													
140–205	All wsites	139.6	9.4	7.5	6.0	8.1	8.8	12.5	18.4	34.5	68.2	120.4	238.6	401.4	631.7	938.9	1195.6	1360.5	1196.0	921.6
	hereof:																			
151 152, 153	stomach	38.8	0.1	0.1	0.1	0.2	0.4	1.1	2.5	7.7	15.1	32.0	72.0	113.9	182.0	278.8	368.9	398.6	322.9	227.8
	intestine except rectum	4.3	0.1	0.1	0.1	0.1	0.3	0.6	0.8	1.5	2.5	4.3	7.2	10.2	18.5	26.7	41.6	48.6	35.2	24.0
154	rectum	3.4	—	0.0	0.0	0.1	0.1	0.3	0.4	1.1	1.4	2.8	6.0	9.7	14.4	24.5	30.8	35.9	36.1	33.4
162, 163	lung	31.8	0.2	0.1	0.1	0.3	0.3	0.6	1.6	5.2	14.3	25.6	56.9	112.2	173.6	250.3	260.3	218.1	142.2	69.0
177	prostate	7.0	0.0	—	0.0	0.0	0.1	0.1	0.1	0.1	0.4	0.8	2.8	7.1	20.0	45.6	92.1	167.4	191.1	181.8
	rate per case	0.002	0.025	0.021	0.018	0.020	0.028	0.032	0.029	0.028	0.033	0.042	0.057	0.045	0.052	0.073	0.125	0.238	0.475	1.045
								FEMALES													
140–205	All sites	124.8	8.2	5.7	4.7	6.0	7.7	12.3	21.7	45.4	80.3	131.8	212.1	282.4	393.4	545.2	730.5	836.2	740.2	613.4
	whereof:																			
151 152, 153	stomach	23.8	0.1	—	0.1	0.1	0.3	1.1	2.1	4.3	8.0	15.1	29.0	43.5	75.1	124.9	182.4	208.1	181.1	132.9
	intestine except rectum	5.2	0.1	0.0	0.0	0.1	0.3	0.3	0.7	1.3	1.9	4.0	7.1	9.6	17.3	24.4	37.1	46.4	38.8	30.1
154	rectum	3.2	0.1	—	—	0.0	0.3	0.2	0.4	0.9	1.6	3.2	4.5	7.3	11.7	13.9	21.6	24.4	17.4	11.4
162, 163	lung	5.9	0.1	0.1	0.0	0.1	0.2	0.3	0.5	1.6	2.5	5.3	10.4	14.3	22.1	32.2	34.6	39.4	28.0	19.9
170	breast	13.2	0.0	—	—	—	0.1	0.9	2.5	7.9	15.0	23.3	33.7	38.9	42.6	46.4	50.1	53.7	57.9	54.9
171	cervix uteri	9.5	—	—	—	0.0	0.1	1.6	4.2	8.3	15.2	20.5	28.1	25.6	27.1	28.7	30.9	27.8	22.2	16.3
172–174	uterus-other and unspecified	9.0	0.0	0.0	0.0	0.2	0.3	0.9	1.6	3.5	8.1	13.2	21.4	25.5	30.8	36.4	42.5	43.8	33.4	22.0
	rate per case	0.002	0.026	0.022	0.019	0.020	0.028	0.032	0.029	0.028	0.029	0.036	0.048	0.038	0.043	0.053	0.080	0.130	0.220	0.406

Table A-8
Poland (urban), 1967-69.
Average annual mortality per 100,000 by age, sex and primary cancer localization

ICD 1955 rev.	Site	Total	0-4	5-9	10-14	15-19	20-24	25-29	30-34	35-39	40-44	45-49	50-54	55-59	60-64	65-69	70-74	75-79	80-84	85+
									MALES											
140-205	All sites whereof:	141.8	9.9	8.0	5.8	7.4	8.5	12.1	18.3	34.2	73.5	134.5	250.8	431.9	700.8	1064.4	1386.8	1617.3	1562.4	1427.4
151	stomach	31.7	0.0	0.2	0.1	0.1	0.4	0.7	2.7	6.7	13.6	30.7	58.2	98.2	160.6	249.6	350.0	345.5	384.4	357.5
152, 153	intestine except rectum	5.2	0.0	0.0	0.1	0.1	0.4	0.3	0.6	1.7	2.7	5.5	9.3	13.7	24.8	35.9	60.2	68.2	55.4	40.3
154	rectum	3.9	—	0.0	0.0	0.2	0.0	0.6	0.5	1.0	1.8	3.4	6.1	10.6	18.9	33.5	36.5	49.4	45.6	61.8
162, 163	lung	37.3	0.0	0.1	0.0	0.2	0.1	0.2	1.9	5.5	17.4	35.6	70.1	137.8	220.6	334.0	355.8	332.8	223.7	123.6
177	prostate	7.3	0.0	—	0.0	0.0	0.1	0.1	0.1	0.1	0.5	0.7	2.9	6.3	21.4	52.7	111.3	205.2	266.0	290.3
Rate per case		0.004	0.056	0.047	0.038	0.037	0.051	0.057	0.052	0.050	0.060	0.082	0.118	0.096	0.116	0.168	0.292	0.555	1.086	2.688
									FEMALES											
140-205	All sites whereof:	135.5	8.5	5.6	4.4	5.4	6.7	13.1	22.5	48.5	86.2	148.5	231.5	303.4	426.4	602.2	797.1	943.6	908.6	797.5
151	stomach	21.3	0.1	—	0.0	—	0.3	0.8	2.2	3.9	6.9	13.8	24.2	35.3	63.5	113.4	161.9	204.5	208.9	151.7
152, 153	intestine, except rectum	6.3	0.2	0.0	—	0.0	0.3	0.5	0.8	1.4	2.1	4.5	8.7	12.5	21.6	28.0	44.4	55.4	56.6	41.7
154	rectum	3.6	—	—	—	—	0.3	0.1	0.4	1.0	1.8	3.2	5.1	8.5	12.6	17.2	25.8	25.8	23.9	11.7
162, 163	lung	6.9	0.1	0.0	—	0.1	0.1	0.2	0.4	1.9	3.1	7.1	12.5	16.7	25.8	38.5	36.3	48.4	37.4	28.3
170	breast	16.2	0.1	—	—	0.2	0.2	1.1	2.7	8.5	16.6	28.9	42.0	47.7	52.0	59.8	62.3	70.4	77.9	85.8
171	cervix uteri	11.4	—	—	—	0.0	0.1	1.8	4.2	10.1	18.7	24.7	30.9	29.6	32.5	36.3	38.2	33.8	30.0	25.8
172-174	uterus-other and unspecified	9.3	0.1	—	—	0.1	0.0	0.9	1.5	3.1	8.1	13.4	20.1	25.3	31.7	41.3	48.8	50.6	42.2	29.2
Rate per case		0.004	0.059	0.049	0.040	0.038	0.049	0.055	0.051	0.050	0.054	0.071	0.095	0.076	0.086	0.107	0.157	0.251	0.435	0.833

Table A-9
Poland (rural), 1967–69.
Average annual mortality per 100,000 by age, sex and primary cancer localization

1955 rev. ICD	Site	Total	0–4	5–9	10–14	15–19	20–24	25–29	30–34	35–39	40–44	45–49	50–54	55–59	60–64	65–69	70–74	75–79	80–84	85+
	MALES																			
140–205	All sites	137.5	8.8	7.0	6.1	9.3	9.2	13.0	18.6	35.0	61.6	113.8	226.9	374.8	575.0	843.2	1051.9	1125.6	910.3	600.0
	whereof:																			
151	stomach	45.6	0.2	0.0	0.0	0.2	0.4	1.7	2.3	9.1	16.9	33.4	85.0	127.7	199.5	301.3	383.0	396.7	275.0	145.3
152, 153	intestine, except rectum	3.3	0.1	0.1	0.1	0.2	0.2	0.4	1.1	1.2	2.3	3.0	5.2	7.2	13.4	19.6	27.6	33.8	19.5	13.7
154	rectum	3.0	—	—	—	0.1	0.2	0.4	0.3	1.1	0.9	2.0	5.8	9.0	10.7	17.6	26.5	25.9	28.8	15.4
162, 163	lung	26.5	0.3	0.1	0.1	0.5	0.4	0.7	1.3	4.8	10.4	23.7	44.4	89.7	135.0	186.0	188.8	139.3	78.7	34.2
177	prostate	6.7	0.0	—	—	0.0	—	0.1	0.1	0.1	0.2	1.0	2.6	7.8	18.8	40.2	77.7	138.9	132.8	112.8
	Rate per case	0.004	0.045	0.039	0.035	0.044	0.061	0.073	0.067	0.065	0.073	0.088	0.112	0.084	0.095	0.129	0.219	0.417	0.846	1.709
140–205	All sites	113.4	7.9	5.7	5.0	6.7	9.1	11.1	20.6	41.3	73.3	113.9	192.3	261.4	360.4	489.2	662.1	720.4	567.6	438.1
	whereof:																			
151	stomach	26.4	0.2	—	0.1	0.2	0.2	1.5	2.0	4.8	9.4	16.3	34.0	51.7	86.7	136.2	203.6	212.0	152.6	115.1
152, 153	intestine, except rectum	4.1	0.0	—	0.1	0.1	0.4	0.1	0.7	1.0	1.7	3.5	5.4	6.6	13.0	20.8	29.7	36.7	20.5	19.0
154	rectum	2.8	0.2	—	—	0.1	0.2	0.2	0.5	0.8	1.4	3.1	3.9	6.1	10.8	10.7	17.3	23.0	10.7	11.1
162, 163	lung	4.9	—	0.1	0.0	—	0.2	0.3	0.6	1.3	1.8	3.4	8.2	11.9	18.5	26.0	32.8	29.7	18.3	11.9
170	breast	10.0	—	—	—	—	0.1	0.5	2.1	7.1	13.2	17.3	25.2	30.1	33.2	33.2	37.5	35.6	37.5	25.4
171	cervix uteri	7.6	—	—	—	—	0.2	1.4	4.1	6.1	11.0	16.0	25.3	21.5	21.7	21.3	23.4	21.3	14.3	7.1
172–174	uterus-other and unspecified	8.5	0.0	0.0	0.0	0.2	0.6	0.8	1.7	3.8	8.2	12.8	22.7	25.6	30.0	31.6	36.0	36.5	24.5	15.1
	Rate per case	0.004	0.047	0.041	0.037	0.044	0.064	0.077	0.070	0.064	0.064	0.076	0.097	0.076	0.086	0.105	0.162	0.270	0.446	0.794

Table A-10

Poland (total country), 1959–61.

Average annual mortality per 100,000 by age, sex and primary cancer localization

ICD 1955 rev.	Site	Total	0–4	5–9	10–14	15–19	20–24	25–29	30–34	35–39	40–44	45–49	50–54	55–59	60–64	65–69	70–74	75–79	80–84	85+
	MALES																			
140–205	All sites	91.4	7.5	5.8	5.1	5.5	9.0	10.9	16.6	26.9	52.2	104.0	187.2	325.6	485.4	680.6	768.9	837.2	806.3	588.8
	whereof:																			
151	stomach	31.9	0.1	0.1	0.2	0.2	0.6	1.5	3.9	7.6	18.5	37.8	65.6	116.4	180.5	259.4	295.0	313,0	273.4	142.8
152, 153	intestine, except rectum	2.2	0.1	0.1	0.1	0.0	0.5	0.2	0.6	0.8	1.9	2.9	4.3	7.8	11.6	15.5	19.4	21.3	23.1	14.3
154	rectum	1.8	0.0	—	—	0.0	0.0	0.1	0.3	0.6	1.0	2.2	2.6	6.9	9.7	12.2	18.5	20.9	21.7	17.5
162, 163	lung	14.5	0.2	0.1	0.1	0.3	0.5	0.8	1.2	2.8	6.3	16.2	35.2	64.9	91.6	117.8	111.7	82.8	56.6	25.4
177	prostate	2.4	0.0	—	—	0.1	—	0.1	—	0.2	0.1	0.7	1.2	3.6	9.3	18.6	40.2	65.1	76.2	61.9
	Rate per case	0.002	0.019	0.019	0.021	0.034	0.039	0.029	0.030	0.035	0.053	0.045	0.042	0.051	0.071	0.113	0.172	0.317	0.699	1.581
	FEMALES																			
140–205	All sites	88.5	6.3	4.3	3.1	4.5	6.3	12.1	22.8	41.8	71.7	125.9	173.9	239.0	324.4	420.8	502.6	570.5	605.8	461.4
	whereof:																			
151	stomach	20.0	0.1	0.1	0.1	0.1	0.3	1.3	3.2	6.1	9.4	19.6	30.4	51.1	81.4	117.8	148.8	167.7	174.8	116.7
152, 153	intestine, except rectum	2.6	0.1	0.0	—	0.1	0.1	0.2	0.5	0.9	1.3	2.8	4.2	6.4	10.4	14.4	17.6	21.6	22.7	19.3
154	rectum	1.7	—	—	—	0.0	0.1	0.2	0.2	0.7	1.4	2.1	3.1	4.5	7.1	8.6	11.5	12.5	11.3	5.3
162, 163	lung	3.5	0.1	0.0	0.1	0.1	0.2	0.4	0.7	1.5	2.1	4.9	7.1	9.5	15.4	22.4	18.9	20.7	13.1	9.3
170	breast	6.2	—	0.0	—	—	0.1	0.4	1.7	3.1	7.9	13.5	17.0	19.7	21.6	24.6	25.3	27.8	27.3	23.3
171	cervix uteri	3.7	—	—	—	0.1	0.2	0.8	2.1	4.6	7.3	9.8	9.6	10.7	10.1	11.9	9.8	10.3	8.5	8.7
172–174	uterus-other and unspecified	8.7	0.0	0.0	0.0	0.1	0.6	1.2	3.3	7.3	11.1	19.2	22.9	26.2	30.9	33.8	33.3	27.8	32.9	24.0
	Rate per case	0.002	0.020	0.019	0.022	0.035	0.031	0.029	0.028	0.030	0.046	0.038	0.037	0.043	0.053	0.077	0.104	0.178	0.355	0.663

Table A-11
Poland (urban) 1959-61.
Average annual mortality per 100,000 by age, sex and primary cancer localization

ICD 1955 rev.	Site	Total	Age																		
			0–4	5–9	10–14	15–19	20–24	25–29	30–34	35–39	40–44	45–49	50–54	55–59	60–64	65–69	70–74	75–79	80–84	85+
			MALES																		
140–205	All sites whereof:	104.1	8.3	6.7	5.9	5.4	7.7	10.5	17.1	29.2	56.3	115.9	217.2	382.2	612.6	892.7	1091.8	1293.4	1262.7	980.1
151	stomach	31.2	0.0	0.1	0.0	0.3	0.2	1.3	3.6	7.9	17.9	36.9	62.6	112.6	188.7	286.6	376.8	441.5	386.2	187.5
152, 153	intestine, except rectum	3.0	0.0	0.1	0.1	0.1	0.5	0.2	0.5	1.1	2.3	4.3	5.8	10.5	16.8	25.7	33.6	33.1	43.1	25.0
154	rectum	2.5	—	—	—	0.1	0.1	0.2	0.5	0.7	1.9	3.1	3.6	10.6	14.5	19.1	31.9	38.5	34.5	33.3
162, 163	lung	20.8	0.3	0.0	0.1	0.2	0.4	1.0	1.5	3.6	8.2	22.9	53.5	100.1	148.9	199.2	196.3	150.8	105.2	54.2
177	prostate	3.5	0.1	—	—	0.2	—	0.1	—	0.1	0.1	1.2	1.7	5.7	14.7	30.6	69.3	114.6	144.8	120.8
	Rate per case	0.005	0.044	0.040	0.048	0.066	0.073	0.054	0.055	0.066	0.110	0.094	0.093	0.118	0.171	0.273	0.415	0.770	1.719	4.076
			FEMALES																		
140–205	All sites whereof:	110.2	6.9	5.2	3.6	4.3	6.0	13.1	26.1	46.6	83.0	148.7	210.7	283.8	409.2	550.1	698.1	807.3	891.0	712.2
151	stomach	21.5	0.0	0.0	—	—	0.2	1.1	3.3	4.6	8.1	17.5	29.3	48.5	86.3	131.5	183.5	219.6	247.4	172.7
152, 153	intestine, except rectum	3.6	0.0	0.0	—	—	0.1	0.2	0.6	1.2	1.9	3.1	5.2	8.4	14.3	20.4	27.5	37.7	34.6	39.4
154	rectum	2.5	—	—	0.1	0.2	0.1	0.2	0.1	1.1	2.0	3.1	4.9	6.3	10.7	12.5	16.9	19.6	21.0	7.6
162, 163	lung	4.7	0.2	0.1	—	—	0.1	0.5	0.8	1.9	2.5	6.4	8.7	13.1	21.3	29.5	29.9	31.7	18.0	13.6
170	breast	9.5	—	—	0.2	—	0.1	0.4	2.5	4.4	11.4	21.3	25.7	29.8	34.5	37.7	42.1	46.8	47.4	40.9
171	cervix uteri	5.6	—	—	—	0.1	0.2	1.1	3.0	6.9	10.7	13.6	15.8	15.9	16.4	17.9	14.5	18.1	11.3	15.1
172–174	uterus-other and unspecified	12.1	—	—	—	0.1	0.7	1.7	4.0	8.6	14.0	25.5	32.2	36.9	43.2	49.2	54.4	41.9	54.9	42.4
	Rate per case	0.004	0.046	0.042	0.049	0.069	0.059	0.054	0.053	0.058	0.093	0.078	0.077	0.092	0.113	0.160	0.220	0.377	0.750	1.495

Table A-12.
Poland (rural), 1959-61.
Average annual mortality per 100,000 by age, sex and primary cancer localization

ICD 1955 rev.	Site	Total	0–4	5–9	10–14	15–19	20–24	25–29	30–34	35–39	40–44	45–49	50–54	55–59	60–64	65–69	70–74	75–79	80–84	85+
										MALES										
140–205	All sites whereof:	80.1	7.1	5.5	4.5	6.5	10.8	11.5	16.1	25.0	48.8	93.8	162.8	282.8	394.5	531.1	541.7	516.7	492.5	346.5
151	stomach	32.7	0.2	0.2	0.3	0.2	1.1	1.8	4.4	7.3	19.0	38.5	68.0	119.3	174.7	240.2	237.2	222.7	196.5	115.4
152, 153	intestine, except rectum	1.6	0.1	0.1	0.0	—	0.4	0.2	0.7	0.4	1.5	1.7	3.0	5.7	7.9	8.3	9.4	12.9	9.4	7.7
154	rectum	1.1	0.1	—	—	—	—	0.1	—	0.4	0.2	1.4	1.8	4.0	6.2	7.3	9.1	8.6	12.9	7.7
162, 163	lung	8.7	0.2	0.1	0.0	0.3	0.5	0.6	0.8	2.0	4.5	10.2	20.1	37.9	50.4	60.6	51.9	35.1	23.5	7.7
177	prostate	1.4	—	—	—	—	—	0.1	—	—	0.1	0.2	0.9	2.1	5.4	10.2	19.6	30.3	29.4	25.6
	Rate per case	0.004	0.035	0.034	0.039	0.072	0.082	0.064	0.065	0.075	0.104	0.086	0.076	0.091	0.123	0.192	0.293	0.540	1.178	2.582
										FEMALES										
140–205	All sites whereof:	68.9	6.2	4.4	3.2	5.3	6.5	11.1	19.5	37.0	60.8	104.9	140.7	199.6	249.6	328.0	327.9	358.5	351.5	256.0
151	stomach	18.5	0.2	0.1	0.2	0.2	0.4	1.4	3.2	7.7	10.6	21.6	31.4	53.5	77.0	105.3	117.8	121.3	110.8	74.4
152, 153	intestine, except rectum	1.6	0.1	0.0	—	0.3	0.2	0.1	0.4	0.7	0.7	2.4	3.3	4.7	6.8	8.8	8.7	7.1	12.2	3.6
154	rectum	0.9	—	—	—	—	—	0.1	0.3	0.2	0.8	1.1	1.6	2.9	3.9	5.0	6.5	6.1	2.7	3.6
162, 163	lung	2.4	0.0	—	—	0.3	0.4	0.2	0.7	1.0	1.7	3.6	5.6	6.3	10.1	15.9	8.9	10.8	8.8	6.1
170	breast	3.1	—	0.0	—	—	0.1	0.4	0.8	1.8	4.4	6.2	9.1	10.6	10.1	12.5	10.3	10.8	9.4	9.7
171	cervix uteri	1.9	—	—	—	—	0.2	0.4	1.1	2.1	3.9	6.1	3.9	5.9	4.6	6.3	5.5	3.4	6.1	3.6
172–174	uterus-other and unspecified	5.6	0.0	0.1	0.0	0.1	0.4	0.6	2.6	5.9	8.3	13.2	14.5	16.6	19.9	19.7	14.3	15.2	13.5	9.7
	Rate per case	0.004	0.036	0.036	0.041	0.071	0.064	0.063	0.060	0.063	0.091	0.074	0.071	0.082	0.100	0.147	0.198	0.338	0.673	1.193

Table A-13

Native white Americans, 1959–61. Average annual mortality per 100,000 by age, sex and primary cancer localization

ICD 1955 rev.	Site	Total	0–14	15–24	25–34	35–44	45–54	55–64	65–74	75–84	85+
						MALES					
140–205	All sites whereof:	137.4	9.4	10.2	18.2	46.6	160.8	431.9	840.1	1350.2	1894.4
151	stomach	10.1	—	0.0	0.5	2.6	10.1	27.9	67.8	133.1	189.4
152, 153	intestine, except rectum	13.0	0.1	0.3	1.0	3.5	12.1	37.3	85.4	160.7	224.7
154	rectum	5.7	0.0	0.1	0.4	1.4	5.9	17.6	38.2	67.0	88.1
162, 163	lung	31.0	0.0	0.1	1.4	9.8	48.5	137.2	201.5	157.2	115.3
177	prostate	13.4	0.0	0.0	0.0	0.1	2.1	18.7	95.6	291.2	523.8
Rate per case		0.0004	0.0014	0.0032	0.0035	0.0033	0.0039	0.0057	0.0093	0.0244	0.1408
						FEMALES					
140–205	All sites whereof:	122.4	7.3	6.2	19.1	65.6	171.4	315.6	515.0	915.7	1325.6
151	stomach	6.2	0.0	0.0	0.5	1.9	5.0	12.3	31.4	72.2	124.5
152, 153	intestine, except rectum	16.0	0.1	0.2	1.0	4.5	15.7	38.7	80.4	166.8	255.1
154	rectum	4.6	0.0	0.1	0.3	1.3	4.9	11.3	22.7	44.6	74.0
162, 163	lung	5.2	0.0	0.0	0.5	3.1	8.7	15.1	23.2	33.8	36.5
170	breast	24.7	—	0.1	3.8	19.4	49.5	70.3	93.4	136.5	208.2
171	cervix uteri	8.0	—	0.1	2.6	9.5	17.0	21.2	26.5	32.5	35.1
172–174	uterus-other and unspecified	5.6	0.0	0.0	0.3	1.8	6.4	17.3	30.4	42.1	54.7
Rate per case		0.0004	0.0014	0.0032	0.0034	0.0032	0.0038	0.0052	0.0076	0.0174	0.0835

Table A-14

Polish-born Americans, 1959–61. Average annual mortality per 100,000 by age, sex and primary cancer localization

ICD 1955 rev.	Site	Total	0–14	15–24	25–34	35–44	45–54	55–64	65–74	75–84	85+
					MALES						
140–205	All sites whereof:	754.0	31.9	5.4	15.0	41.4	147.3	545.3	1253.0	1800.1	1902.9
151	stomach	98.1	—	5.4	—	8.6	18.9	69.1	161.5	240.3	247.0
152, 153	intestine, except rectum	83.9	—	—	2.1	1.7	12.9	57.3	138.7	211.8	283.6
154	rectum	37.7	—	—	—	0.9	8.0	29.9	57.7	92.7	137.2
162, 163	lung	172.6	—	—	—	6.1	27.4	128.1	323.2	323.7	219.6
177	prostate	58.6	—	—	—	—	1.0	22.8	85.7	227.4	320.2
Rate per case		0.090	15.933	5.356	2.142	0.865	0.497	0.421	0.277	0.917	9.150
					FEMALES						
140–205	All sites whereof:	484.1	16.3	10.0	17.3	83.0	207.8	432.8	667.3	1051.4	1414.0
151	stomach	55.7	—	—	—	6.9	12.5	36.0	80.7	158.1	242.0
152, 153	intestine, except rectum	72.4	—	—	—	4.0	18.2	60.7	102.1	178.1	310.0
154	rectum	22.4	—	—	—	—	6.8	19.2	34.0	50.5	52.9
162, 163	lung	22.2	—	—	3.9	4.0	7.4	17.5	34.3	43.8	60.5
170	breast	57.6	—	—	1.9	24.7	54.6	61.8	60.0	103.8	151.2
171	cervix uteri	16.4	—	—	1.9	7.9	10.8	17.5	21.4	22.9	22.7
172–174	uterus-other and unspecified	22.2	—	—	—	—	8.5	25.7	33.2	31.4	37.8
Rate per case		0.088	16.323	4.968	1.943	0.989	0.569	0.343	0.268	0.952	7.562

Table A-15

Polish-born Americans, 1950. Average annual mortality per 100,000 by age, sex and primary cancer localization

ICD 1955 rev.	Site	Age								
		Total	0–14	15–24	25–34	35–44	45–54	55–64	65–74	75+
		MALES								
140–205	All sites whereof:	624.8	—	19.2	13.6	59.8	212.9	706.2	1140.5	1510.9
151	stomach	121.2	—	—	—	10.0	60.6	124.4	222.0	361.9
152, 153	intestine, except rectum	50.8	—	—	—	—	22.7	57.9	93.4	126.4
154	rectum	32.6	—	—	—	5.0	15.2	34.0	65.8	68.9
162, 163	lung	127.4	—	—	6.8	7.5	42.4	163.0	235.8	212.6
177	prostate	36.7	—	—	—	—	6.1	29.4	78.1	183.8
Rate per case		0.34		19.2	6.8	2.494	1.515	0.773	1.531	5.747
		FEMALES								
140–205	All sites whereof:	380.7	—	16.8	31.2	96.8	245.2	425.2	667.4	994.2
151	stomach	53.3	—	—	—	5.0	25.0	47.3	129.5	173.7
152, 153	intestine, except rectum	43.0	—	—	—	7.4	35.0	44.7	65.6	143.7
154	rectum	22.7	—	—	6.2	2.5	10.0	21.9	45.6	89.8
162, 163	lung	16.3	—	—	—	—	6.3	23.7	25.5	47.9
170	breast	50.8	—	—	6.2	19.9	53.8	60.5	49.2	119.8
171	cervix uteri	21.5	—	—	—	9.9	25.0	26.3	23.7	24.0
172–174	uterus-other and unspecified	22.4	—	—	—	5.0	17.5	26.3	43.8	24.0
Rate per case		0.33		16.8	6.2	2.481	1.251	0.876	1.825	5.988

Table A-16
Polish migrants in Australia, 1962—66.
Average annual mortality per 100,000 by age, sex and primary cancer localization

ICD, 1955 rev.	Site	Total	0–9	10–19	20–29	30–39	40–49	50–59	60–69	70–79	80–89	90+
								MALES				
140–205	All sites	147.1	—	15.6	—	30.6	75.5	229.6	568.5	1502.8	2479.5	—
	whereof:											
151	stomach	32.4	—	—	—	8.3	23.4	44.6	124.1	225.4	551.0	—
152, 153	intestine, except rectum	6.0	—	—	—	—	2.7	2.3	41.4	112.7	275.5	—
154	rectum	4.9	—	—	—	—	1.4	9.4	10.3	112.7	—	—
162, 163	lung	37.3	—	—	—	2.8	9.6	58.6	227.5	413.2	551.0	—
177	prostate	4.4	—	—	—	—	1.4	2.3	31.0	75.1	275.5	—
Rate per case		0.549	59.101	15.617	10.035	2.781	1.375	2.346	10.339	37.565	275.48	5000.0
								FEMALES				
140–205	All sites	154.8	—	—	9,1	40.0	95.1	242.0	634.3	939.7	1854.9	1666.7
	whereof:											
151	stomach	21.2	—	—	—	6.1	14.2	34.5	59.8	134.2	463.7	—
152, 153	intestine, except rectum	11.4	—	—	—	—	2.4	28.8	24.0	134.2	309.1	—
154	rectum	4.1	—	—	—	—	—	11.5	23.9	33.6	—	—
162, 163	lung	8.2	—	—	—	—	9.5	5.8	35.9	33.6	154.6	—
170	breast	23.7	—	—	—	3.1	19.0	57.6	95.7	67.1	—	—
171	cervix uteri	9.0	—	—	—	9.2	9.5	17.3	—	33.6	—	—
172–174	uterus-other and unspecified	4.9	—	—	—	—	2.4	5.8	12.0	33.6	154.6	—
Rate per case		0.816	61.690	17.088	9.111	3.071	2.371	5.756	11.958	33.557	154.55	1666.6

Table A-17

Age-adjusted cancer mortality rates in Poland, in the United States, and in Polish migrants. Brackets show the 95 percent confidence limits. Standard —,world population"[41]

Sex	ICD, 155 rev.	Site	Poland		Native white Americans 1959–1961	Polish migrants		
			1967–1969	1959–1961		US 1959–1961	US 1950	Australia 1962–1966
Males	140–205	All sites	148.9 (147.7–150.1)	108.9 (107.8–110.0)	136.7 (136.2–137.2)	176.9 (162.1–191.7)	186.1 (176.0–196.2)	145.2 (120.1–170.3)
		whereof:						
	151	stomach	41.5 (40.8–42.2)	38.3 (37.6–39.0)	10.1 (10.0–10.2)	22.5 (20.1–24.9)	36.2 (32.4–40.0)	28.8 (17.7–39.9)
	152, 153	intestine, except rectum	4.6 (4.4–4.8)	2.7 (2.5–2.9)	12.8 (12.6–13.0)	18.0 (16.5–19.5)	14.3 (12.0–16.6)	9.6 (3.5–15.7)
	154	rectum	3.7 (3.5–3.9)	2.2 (2.0–2.4)	5.6 (5.5–5.7)	5.6 (4.6–6.6)	9.7 (7.7–11.7)	5.1 (0–10.5)
	162, 163	lung	33.2 (32.6–33.8)	16.8 (16.4–17.2)	30.7 (30.5–30.9)	40.5 (38.6–42.4)	35.6 (31.5–39.7)	40.6 (26.0–55.2)
	177	prostate	8.1 (7.8–8.4)	3.4 (3.2–3.6)	13.5 (13.3–13.7)	11.2 (10.2–12.2)	10.6 (8.6–12.6)	7.6 (0.7–14.5)

Table A-17 continued

Sex	ICD, 1955 rev.	Site	Poland		Native white Americans 1959-1961	Polish migrants		
			1967-1969	1959-1961		US 1959-1961	US 1950	Australia 1962-1966
Females	140-205	All sites	104.6 (103.5-105.7)	84.0 (83.0-85.0)	105.6 (105.2-106.0)	133.1 (121.7-144.5)	133.1 (123.1-143.1)	147.3 (124.8-169.8)
	151	whereof: stomach	19.1 (18.7-19.5)	18.9 (18.5-19.3)	5.1 (5.0-5.2)	12.7 (11.5-13.9)	17.1 (14.4-19.8)	18.4 (10.1-26.7)
	152, 153	intestine, except rectum	4.3 (4.1-4.5)	2.5 (2.4-2.6)	13.4 (13.3-13.5)	16.7 (15.3-18.1)	14.5 (11.9-17.1)	11.7 (4.9-18.5)
	154	rectum	2.6 (2.4-2.8)	1.6 (1.5-1.7)	3.8 (3.7-3.9)	5.0 (4.3-5.7)	8.1 (6.6-9.6)	3.7 (0.3-3.9)
	162, 163	lung	4.9 (4.7-5.1)	3.3 (3.1-3.5)	4.4 (4.3-4.5)	6.9 (5.7-8.1)	4.8 (3.5-6.1)	6.7 (0.7-12.7)
	170	breast	11.4 (11.0-11.8)	5.9 (5.7-6.1)	21.7 (21.5-21.9)	19.5 (17.5-21.5)	18.9 (15.4-22.4)	16.5 (8.3-24.7)
	171	cervix uteri	8.5 (8.2-8.8)	3.6 (3.4-3.8)	11.8 (11.7-11.9)	10.6 (10.0-11.2)	15.0 (12.4-17.6)	25.7 (15.7-35.7)
	172-174	uterus-other and unspecified	7.8 (7.5-8.1)	8.3 (8.1-8.5)				

Table A-18
Standardized mortality ratios, SMR, by sex, district of residence, and primary cancer site in 1967–1969 in Poland.
Brackets show the 95 percent confidence limits.
SMR = 100 for all inhabitants of Poland of the same sex and at the same timeperiod

ICD, 1955 rev.	Site	City						Białystok	Byd-goszcz	Gdańsk	Kato-wice
		Warsza-wa	Kraków	Łódź	Poznań	Wrocław	Total, 5 metropo-litan cities				
											M A
140–205	All sites	117	114	129	111	120	119	78	110	109	113
		(110–124)	(107–121)	(121–137)	(104–118)	(112–127)	(112–126)	(73–83)	(103–117)	(102–115)	(106–12
	whereof:										
151	stomach	78	85	99	92	86	87	95	103	97	104
		(72–84)	(74–98)	(90–108)	(81–104)	(74–100)	(82–92)	(88–103)	(97–109)	(89–105)	(98–11
152, 153	intestine,	181	156	162	158	150	167	55	108	97	138
	except rectum	(152–214)	(115–206)	(128–202)	(117–209)	(103–208)	(149–185)	(40–74)	(89–130)	(76–123)	(123–15
154	rectum	84	177	131	123	128	118	83	94	110	163
		(62–111)	(129–237)	(97–173)	(82–176)	(80–192)	(103–136)	(64–108)	(76–116)	(86–140)	(145–18
162, 163	lung	146	163	141	114	147	143	58	115	125	123
		(137–156)	(145–181)	(128–154)	(100–129)	(129–166)	(134–152)	(52–64)	(108–122)	(116–135)	(116–13
177	prostate	134	102	119	143	133	127	81	118	132	116
		(114–157)	(74–137)	(96–147)	(111–182)	(94–181)	(116–140)	(67–97)	(103–136)	(111–156)	(106–12
											F E M
140–205	All sites	119	113	130	123	109	120	79	114	107	111
		(112–126)	(106–120)	(122–138)	(116–130)	(102–115)	(113–127)	(74–84)	(107–121)	(101–113)	(104–11
	whereof:										
151	stomach	73	91	101	89	86	85	107	99	95	105
		(66–80)	(78–105)	(90–112)	(76–103)	(71–103)	(80–90)	(97–116)	(92–107)	(85–104)	(99–11
152, 153	intestine,	148	138	128	161	118	141	70	103	103	141
	except rectum	(129–170)	(108–175)	(101–160)	(126–204)	(84–160)	(128–154)	(55–89)	(87–120)	(83–128)	(128–15
154	rectum	93	135	143	151	147	123	73	85	110	144
		(72–118)	(96–184)	(111–182)	(107–205)	(97–213)	(108–139)	(53–98)	(67–106)	(85–143)	(127–16
162, 163	lung	177	140	105	138	122	145	72	96	126	101
		(156–200)	(111–175)	(85–130)	(107–175)	(87–166)	(132–158)	(57–90)	(82–112)	(105–151)	(90–11
170	breast	152	143	144	173	122	148	92	121	111	115
		(138–166)	(119–166)	(128–161)	(149–201)	(100–149)	(139–157)	(79–107)	(110–132)	(98–125)	(108–12
171–174	uterus	89	107	109	109	107	101	63	119	116	118
		(81–98)	(92–124)	(97–122)	(92–127)	(89–128)	(95–107)	(55–72)	(109–128)	(104–128)	(111–12

					District								
...ielce	Koszalin	Kraków	Lublin	Łódź	Olsztyn	Opole	Poznań	Rzeszów	Szczecin	Warsza-wa	Wrocław	Zielona Góra
...S												
96	109	99	81	96	99	104	98	91	104	97	105	99
(0–102)	(103–115)	(93–105)	(76–86)	(90–102)	(94–105)	(98–110)	(92–104)	(85–96)	(98–110)	(91–103)	(99–111)	(93–105)
122	115	112	77	101	114	102	110	108	94	103	95	98
5–129)	(102–128)	(105–119)	(72–82)	(95–107)	(104–124)	(93–111)	(103–117)	(101–114)	(84–105)	(97–108)	(88–101)	(88–109)
74	81	95	70	92	79	91	103	74	84	86	103	112
1–90)	(54–117)	(79–114)	(57–87)	(76–110)	(55–110)	(67–120)	(87–120)	(60–92)	(56–120)	(72–101)	(83–128)	(83–148)
54	114	97	78	110	72	126	95	83	87	95	101	94
2–70)	(76–163)	(79–118)	(63–97)	(90–134)	(47–105)	(97–164)	(78–116)	(66–104)	(56–128)	(79–114)	(79–128)	(63–134)
80	116	93	80	81	95	112	87	83	147	85	108	124
4–86)	(103–130)	(86–99)	(74–86)	(75–87)	(84–106)	(102–122)	(81–92)	(77–89)	(134–162)	(80–90)	(100–116)	(112–136)
87	102	84	85	86	89	115	126	88	115	97	89	70
5–100)	(75–135)	(73–97)	(73–99)	(74–100)	(68–116)	(95–138)	(112–141)	(75–103)	(88–149)	(85–110)	(74–107)	(51–94)
LES												
93	102	94	77	99	91	101	103	95	103	93	107	101
7–99)	(96–108)	(88–100)	(72–82)	(93–105)	(85–96)	(95–107)	(97–109)	(89–101)	(97–109)	(87–98)	(101–113)	(95–107)
120	97	123	72	98	116	104	101	127	98	91	108	107
12–127)	(83–112)	(116–130)	(65–78)	(91–105)	(103–130)	(93–116)	(95–107)	(118–136)	(85–113)	(85–97)	(98–118)	(94–123)
79	95	101	63	84	87	103	114	74	85	68	106	103
56–95)	(67–129)	(87–117)	(52–77)	(70–101)	(64–115)	(82–129)	(99–131)	(61–90)	(60–116)	(57–80)	(88–127)	(76–136)
58	67	99	84	74	92	127	94	123	84	92	108	83
45–75)	(39–107)	(81–121)	(68–104)	(58–94)	(62–132)	(98–165)	(78–115)	(101–150)	(54–125)	(76–110)	(84–137)	(54–122)
85	108	87	91	78	99	100	77	98	131	93	116	120
72–99)	(80–142)	(75–101)	(77–106)	(65–92)	(76–129)	(81–124)	(65–90)	(83–115)	(102–166)	(81–107)	(97–137)	(94–152)
76	79	82	66	101	67	105	121	78	83	88	90	74
58–85)	(64–98)	(73–91)	(58–75)	(92–111)	(54–82)	(91–121)	(111–131)	(69–87)	(68–101)	(80–97)	(80–101)	(61–90)
85	118	86	72	91	108	114	110	94	125	81	130	124
77–93)	(103–136)	(78–94)	(65–79)	(83–91)	(93–124)	(101–128)	(102–118)	(85–102)	(109–146)	(74–87)	(118–142)	(109–140)

Table A-19

Population of Poland on December 31, 1967, by sex, age, and district of residence[219] A. Males

District	Total	0-4	5-9	10-14	15-19	20-24	25-29	30-34	35-39	40-44	45-49	50-54	55-59	60-64	65-69	70+
Poland (all districts)	15,577,104	1,306,510	1,597,145	1,805,649	1,663,720	1,138,465	1,058,405	1,144,993	1,189,142	1,000,465	744,637	606,269	750,301	630,286	446,634	494,483
Warszawa City	583,724	30,049	42,671	60,914	57,732	44,504	36,137	47,693	58,690	51,686	33,904	25,126	32,389	26,498	17,056	18,675
Kraków City	265,212	16,202	20,213	25,381	30,549	28,458	19,830	21,889	23,596	20,028	13,615	10,453	12,620	9,551	6,083	6,744
Łódź City	344,538	18,322	25,161	35,477	37,199	28,344	21,236	24,489	29,146	30,000	21,955	16,459	19,261	16,008	10,528	10,953
Poznań City	212,079	12,447	16,245	21,967	24,648	19,690	13,880	14,997	16,152	14,943	11,480	9,601	12,018	9,797	6,441	7,773
Wrocław City	244,784	14,591	20,070	27,080	32,009	23,488	17,945	20,063	22,333	20,876	14,070	8,762	8,494	6,184	4,310	4,509
Białystok D.	570,414	52,740	62,789	66,565	54,737	36,207	37,203	39,571	43,658	34,728	24,205	19,498	28,685	26,138	19,505	24,185
Bydgoszcz D.	909,988	80,269	97,668	111,429	103,923	66,390	58,657	61,492	63,235	52,758	40,327	35,186	44,626	38,282	25,526	30,220
Gdańsk D.	703,364	61,464	74,159	84,942	82,189	53,215	51,633	54,958	54,267	42,625	31,142	25,698	30,149	24,277	15,845	16,801
Katowice D.	1,752,073	135,958	162,445	174,088	179,736	137,754	156,050	149,445	145,145	106,432	76,887	67,731	83,838	70,334	51,293	54,937
Kielce D.	916,033	76,877	96,070	112,529	92,918	61,799	52,085	59,212	64,745	59,022	46,596	41,586	48,783	39,922	29,810	34,079
Koszalin D.	380,806	36,630	47,179	52,059	44,533	26,748	24,759	27,608	29,094	23,166	16,833	12,870	13,446	10,591	7,607	7,683
Kraków D.	1,047,913	102,000	115,028	118,807	101,489	71,936	68,325	75,851	74,752	62,991	47,146	40,089	53,208	46,490	34,499	35,302
Lublin D.	933,769	76,148	91,462	105,918	92,746	64,829	58,401	63,250	70,494	62,413	47,784	39,844	50,331	42,977	30,857	36,315
Łódź D.	810,034	63,199	77,612	90,759	82,694	59,638	49,373	53,585	55,722	51,314	42,574	37,634	46,000	37,976	28,128	33,826
Olsztyn D.	479,801	50,586	61,935	63,468	51,831	31,542	33,578	36,871	36,740	27,066	19,140	14,194	16,831	14,712	10,199	11,108
Opole D.	492,116	49,657	58,078	53,980	49,171	31,062	40,423	44,473	40,907	26,032	18,427	14,086	19,368	18,027	13,180	15,245
Poznań D.	1,042,266	92,409	109,752	122,343	113,250	75,556	64,018	67,840	67,881	59,549	49,661	44,322	57,623	48,192	31,698	38,172
Rzeszów D.	833,988	80,328	90,780	94,297	82,498	54,521	52,301	58,649	59,572	51,566	37,529	30,457	45,219	39,963	28,919	27,389
Szczecin D.	436,818	37,166	47,473	57,035	52,820	34,666	30,893	34,295	36,098	30,834	20,963	14,269	13,962	10,937	7,647	7,760
Warszawa D.	1,227,430	99,958	122,472	142,446	128,458	89,644	82,182	86,385	89,641	78,595	60,355	49,191	61,449	52,860	39,336	44,458
Wrocław D.	964,142	81,153	108,990	127,812	117,886	67,754	62,081	71,731	74,878	66,949	49,681	34,334	35,712	27,466	18,889	18,826
Zielona Góra D.	425,812	38,357	48,893	56,353	50,704	30,720	27,415	30,646	32,396	26,892	20,363	14,879	16,289	13,104	9,278	9,523

B. Females

District	Total	0-4	5-9	10-14	15-19	20-24	25-29	30-34	35-39	40-44	45-49	50-54	55-59	60-64	65-69	70+
Poland (all districts)	16,509,928	1,246,113	1,524,151	1,730,427	1,615,573	1,144,855	1,048,149	1,132,193	1,197,226	1,137,754	861,793	723,852	880,016	764,057	618,799	884,970
Warszawa City	679,496	28,407	40,583	58,472	55,051	45,678	43,170	54,987	61,074	55,429	40,009	34,416	43,708	38,827	31,051	48,634
Kraków City	286,505	15,488	19,379	24,529	27,068	25,001	18,708	22,174	23,939	21,315	16,198	13,961	16,348	13,933	11,418	17,046
Łódź City	399,974	17,221	23,953	33,528	36,735	29,522	22,968	27,210	34,583	36,269	25,618	20,153	25,308	22,498	17,630	26,778
Poznań City	240,213	12,027	15,478	21,196	23,530	20,856	14,952	16,502	17,369	17,365	13,675	11,941	15,190	13,153	11,057	15,922
Wrocław City	259,558	13,803	19,124	26,139	30,027	23,486	19,012	21,447	23,865	23,808	14,409	9,537	9,918	8,572	7,020	9,391
Białystok. D.	598,999	49,997	59,684	63,702	55,240	38,187	36,537	38,513	43,108	39,165	27,965	24,678	31,840	28,634	24,282	37,467
Bydgoszcz D.	966,607	77,110	93,564	106,267	100,627	66,978	57,828	60,290	63,611	60,477	47,981	43,414	52,514	45,405	36,252	54,289
Gdańsk D.	716,516	59,151	69,853	80,729	76,620	51,070	49,051	52,288	52,331	49,077	36,462	29,037	33,450	27,581	20,827	28,989
Katowice D.	1,827,364	129,378	154,660	166,067	157,597	127,724	140,813	134,182	134,570	124,419	98,255	87,790	106,439	91,104	72,268	102,098
Kielce D.	975,138	73,320	91,940	107,524	94,457	62,338	53,604	60,434	67,507	65,719	53,154	48,225	54,654	46,573	39,427	56,262
Koszalin D.	388,194	35,013	44,831	50,018	43,810	26,989	24,634	27,839	28,384	26,758	18,259	13,167	14,480	12,213	9,594	12,205
Kraków D.	1,118,881	97,304	110,661	114,295	102,079	74,191	68,720	74,859	77,326	71,390	55,525	48,749	61,198	55,542	46,453	60,589
Lublin D.	990,789	73,185	87,828	101,884	93,281	67,897	58,322	61,616	69,935	68,893	54,958	46,863	57,151	49,697	40,181	59,098
Łódź D.	864,083	60,221	74,193	87,239	83,564	60,581	49,511	53,508	58,228	57,744	48,534	43,736	51,359	44,115	36,549	55,001
Olsztyn D.	490,286	48,239	58,607	60,330	51,789	32,032	32,635	35,407	35,615	30,515	21,341	16,217	19,120	16,662	13,357	18,420
Opole D.	532,452	47,275	55,135	51,854	47,278	32,670	40,481	42,981	39,131	34,607	25,173	19,803	26,108	23,388	19,324	27,244
Poznań D.	1,105,323	88,619	105,007	117,652	111,500	75,885	62,502	66,613	68,831	67,595	55,863	52,112	65,399	55,923	43,819	68,003
Rzeszów D.	894,644	76,213	86,890	91,572	82,142	56,509	53,784	59,854	61,727	58,139	45,396	36,094	52,206	47,646	39,540	46,932
Szczecin D.	438,636	35,119	45,532	54,561	50,948	32,317	28,775	33,713	35,296	33,741	21,193	14,188	15,644	13,429	10,644	13,536
Warszawa D.	1,289,554	95,096	116,344	136,925	125,691	92,318	79,479	81,898	88,414	84,685	67,737	58,470	70,245	61,925	51,006	79,321
Wrocław D.	1,006,086	77,258	104,331	121,949	115,960	71,154	64,860	74,342	79,818	79,314	52,446	35,533	39,621	32,123	25,299	32,078
Zielona Góra D.	440,630	36,669	46,574	53,995	50,579	31,472	27,803	31,536	32,564	31,330	21,642	15,768	18,116	15,114	11,801	15,667

Table A-20

Number of physicians and hospital beds per 10,000 population in 1960 and 1969; percentage of deaths certified by physicians, and number of deaths certified as due to senility and other ill-defined conditions (Nos. 780 = 795, ICD, 1955 rev.) in 1960 and 1967; length of roads with hard surface dressing, per 100 square kilometers, in 1960 and 1969 in Poland, by districts

	Year (reference source)	CITY						DISTRICT																
		Poland	Warszawa	Kraków	Łódź	Poznań	Wrocław	Białystok	Bydgoszcz	Gdańsk	Katowice	Kielce	Koszalin	Kraków	Lublin	Łódź	Olsztyn	Opole	Poznań	Rzeszów	Szczecin	Warszawa	Wrocław	Zielona Góra
Physicians (except dentists) per 10,000 population	1960 (139)	9.6	39.4	34.6	23.5	20.9	21.9	6.7	5.9	13.5	10.0	4.8	6.8	5.8	6.8	6.0	5.9	7.6	6.1	5.4	11.8	5.6	7.7	7.2
	1969 (139)	14.5	50.3	40.4	30.9	36.5	30.1	13.8	10.0	19.5	14.1	8.5	11.3	10.1	10.9	9.1	10.3	11.9	8.2	8.5	18.6	10.3	11.1	11.5
Hospital beds per 10,000 population	1960 (139)	45.3	81.2	109.0	68.3	76.1	87.5	34.1	38.5	55.6	59.9	22.1	55.6	24.0	34.6	26.1	48.1	59.9	35.1	32.1	59.4	24.4	62.1	50.6
	1969 (139)	51.2	91.7	95.4	79.3	84.1	86.2	44.1	41.0	54.0	69.8	30.0	55.1	30.9	42.8	38.6	48.4	62.2	38.5	39.4	54.1	32.5	65.6	52.5
Percent of deaths certified by physicians	1960 (186)	74.6	100.0	100.0	100.0	100.0	100.0	60.1	80.0	89.1	95.1	53.4	77.5	51.0	51.8	73.6	67.4	88.6	81.4	52.7	83.7	65.2	83.9	78.7
	1967 (141)	90.1	99.8	99.8	99.0	99.9	98.9	83.8	90.1	94.9	96.0	82.8	88.6	95.2	84.6	89.2	82.9	89.8	89.8	82.3	87.1	88.5	86.7	85.8
Number of deaths due to "senility and other ill — defined conditions"	1960 (141)	45413	347	285	563	205	120	2908	2677	1169	3792	1616	702	4161	4310	3660	1338	1473	3693	3971	717	5444	1532	730
	1967 (141)	27625	425	194	622	296	112	1438	1746	808	2665	1467	301	1858	2923	1963	751	975	2753	1652	445	2640	1027	564
Length of roads per 100 square kilometers	1960 (138)	33.6						21.0	30.7	40.0	41.8	29.4	37.5	37.0	16.9	36.7	36.7	52.3	39.2	25.1	36.1	25.5	56.8	38.9
	1969 (139)	41.2						29.0	40.9	43.3	51.8	47.0	38.4	52.3	26.4	48.4	37.4	54.0	44.0	37.7	39.6	36.9	56.9	39.8

Table A-21

Cancer of selected sites, and percentage of carcinomas, in the autopsy material of the Pathology Department of Jagiellonian University, 1851–1938[28], and in the incidence data* of Katowice District Register, 1965[183]

ICD, 1955 rev.	Site	Males				Females			
		Total number of cancers		whereof carcinomas (percent)		Total number of cancers		whereof carcinomas (percent)	
		A	I	A	I	A	I	A	I
140–205	Total whereof:	2996	803	81.8	83.3	2851	1515	84.8	89.0
151	stomach	1180	122	99.8	100.0	790	58	99.6	96.5
152, 153	intestine except rectum	117	22	81.8	100.0	92	31	93.5	100.0
154	rectum	117	30	95.7	96.7	87	30	100.0	96.7
162, 163	lung	127	127	91.3	92.1	44	15	81.9	73.3
170	breast	5	—	100.0	—	124	218	96.8	95.4
171–174	uterus	—	—	—	—	689	647	96.8	96.5
177	prostate	24	12	87.5	91.7	—	—	—	—

A Autopsy material, Jagiellonian University.
I Incidence data, Katowice District.

* Limited to cases with the histopathology diagnosis (a little over 50 percent of the reported cancer cases lacked that diagnosis).

Table A-22
The average annual consumption per capita of selected food items in Poland, 1938–1971-in kilograms and expressed as a percentage of consumption in 1938. Source: [140].

YEAR		1938	1946	1947	1948	1949	1950	1951	1952	1953	1954	1955	1956	1957
Potatoes	kg	260	310	305	302	290	270	255	250	245	235	229	235	234
	%	100	119.2	117.3	116.2	111.5	103.8	98.1	96.2	94.2	90.4	88.1	90.4	90.0
Meat	kg	16.5	15.8	21.1	21.7	28.0	36.5	36.7	32.7	35.2	36.2	37.7	41.0	43.9
	%	100	95.8	127.9	131.5	169.7	221.2	222.4	198.2	213.3	219.4	228.5	248.5	266.1
Fats	kg	5.7	3.9	5.0	5.9	7.3	9.7	9.9	9.6	9.8	10.4	11.1	11.9	12.2
	%	100	68.4	87.7	103.5	128.1	170.2	173.7	168.4	171.9	182.5	194.7	208.8	214.0
Sugar	kg	9.6	...	12.8	17.1	19.3	21.0	24.9	22.4	19.9	22.4	24.0	25.2	26.5
	%	100	...	133.3	178.1	201.0	218.8	259.4	233.3	207.3	233.3	250.0	262.5	276.0

YEAR		1958	1959	1960	1961	1962	1963	1964	1965	1966	1967	1968	1969	1970	1971
Potatoes	kg	232	226	223	223	221	218	217	215	211	207	201	199	197	189
	%	89.2	86.9	85.8	85.8	85.0	83.8	83.5	82.7	81.2	79.6	77.3	76.5	75.8	72.7
Meat	kg	45.3	44.1	42.5	45.2	45.8	46.3	47.1	49.2	51.0	52.3	52.2	52.6	52.6	56.2
	%	274.5	267.3	257.6	273.9	277.6	280.6	285,5	298.2	309.1	317.0	316.4	318.8	318.8	340.6
Fats	kg	12.8	13.0	13.6	13.8	14.1	14.3	14.9	15.1	15.4	15.8	16.9	17.5	17.8	18.0
	%	224.6	228.1	238.6	242.1	247.4	250.9	261.4	264.9	270.2	277.2	296.5	307.0	312.3	315.8
Sugar	kg	28.5	29.6	27.9	30.6	30.2	32.3	31.4	32.6	34.1	35.5	36.7	37.2	38.9	39.6
	%	296.9	308.3	290.6	318.8	314.6	336.5	327.1	339.6	355.2	369.8	382.3	387.5	405.2	412.5

Summary

Cancer mortality for the most frequent primary sites, stomach, intestinal tract, lung, breast, uterus and prostate, in Poland in 1959–1969 was analyzed and compared with cancer incidence registered in the selected regions of Poland, with cancer mortality and incidence in other countries, and with cancer mortality in Polish-born migrants to the United States for 1950 and 1959–61, and to Australia for 1962–66.

In comparison with other countries, Poland is characterized by a low, but increasing risk of cancer of the intestinal tract, breast, corpus uteri and prostate. The risk of cancer of the stomach and of uterine cervix in Poland is high; but in recent years the stomach, and possibly uterine cervix, cancer risk have showed some decline. The increase in lung cancer risk is similar in Poland to the increase in other countries.

In 1950, stomach cancer mortality among Polish-born Americans was as high as in Poland; ten years later it had decreased, but was still much above the low rates prevailing for natives of the host country. The intestinal tract cancer mortality of these migrants has risen to the much higher risk prevailing for native Americans. Mortality from cancer of the breast, uterine corpus and prostate among these Polish migrants to the United States has also increased from the low level reported for Poland, but has not yet reached the high level characteristic of the United States. On the other hand, lung cancer mortality among Polish-born Americans was higher than either in Poland or among native Americans.

Displacements in cancer mortality, noted among Polish migrants to Australia, were similar to those for Polish-born Americans.

Geographical differences and time trends in cancer occurrence, exemplified by the data presented for Poland and Polish migrants, point to the primary importance of environmental factors in cancer etiopathogenesis.

Dietary habits and nutrition seem to play an important and similar part in the etiopathogenesis of cancer of the intestinal tract, breast, uterine corpus, and prostate; for stomach cancer they are also probably as important, but the mechanism of their action is likely to be quite different. Uterine cervix cancer seems to depend on infectious, possibly viral factors. The association between lung cancer and cigarette smoking is known quite well, but smoking is not the sole environmental factor in lung cancer etiopathogenesis.

In consideration of the analysis of the results presented, the continuation and extension of studies on the epidemiology of the cancers discussed is justified, and the especially favorable conditions for such studies in Poland and in Polish migrants are stressed. Directions and methods of epidemiologic studies, which are most likely to lead to the identification of carcinogenic factors and, in turn, should permit successful cancer prevention, are discussed.

References

1. Abou-Doud K. T.: Epidemiology of carcinoma of the cervix uteri in Lebanese Christians and Moslems. *Cancer* 20, 1706, 1967.
2. Acheson E. D.: *Record Linkage in Medicine.* Oxford University Press, London, 1967.
3. Ackerman L. V., Spratt J. S. Jr.: Do adenomatous polyps become cancer? *Gastroenterology* 44, 905, 1963.
4. Aitken-Swan J., Baird D.: Circumcision and cancer of the cervix. *Brit. J. Cancer* 19, 217, 1965.
5. Akazaki K.: *The pathology of prostatic cancer. Symposium on prostatic adenoma and cancer. The 16th General Assembly of the Japan Medical Congress.* Osaka, 1963.
6. Apt A.: Circumcision and prostatic cancer. *Acta Med. Scand.* 178, 493, 1965.
7. Arffmann E.: Heated fats and allied compounds as carcinogens: A critical review of experimental results. *J. Nat. Cancer Inst.* 25, 893, 1960.
8. Aries V., Crowther J. S., Drasar B. S., Hill M. J., Williams R. E. O.: Bacteria and the aetiology of cancer of the large bowel. *GUT*, 10, 334, 1969.
9. Ashley D. J. B.: On the incidence of carcinoma of the prostate. *J. Path. Bact.* 90, 217, 1965.
10. Ashley D. J. B.: Environmental factors in the aetiology of gastric cancer. *Brit. J. Prev. Soc. Med.* 23, 187, 1969.
11. Ashley D. J. B.: A male-female differential in tumour incidence. *Brit. J. Cancer* 23, 21, 1969.
12. Ashley D. J. B.: A systematic sex difference in intestinal carcinoma. *Cancer* 25, 966, 1970.
13. Bailar J. C., III: The incidence of independent tumors among uterine cancer patients. *Cancer* 16, 842, 1963.
14. Bailar J. C. III, King H., Mason M. J.: *Cancer Rates and Risks.* Public Health Service Publication No. 1148, Washington, 1964.
15. Beffinger J.: personal information, 1967.
16. Berg J.: Some intercountry and intergroup differences in histological types of cancer. *J. Chron. Dis.* 23, 325, 1970.
17. Bielecki J., Piekutowska B.: Chorzy i zmarli na nowotwory w Polsce w okresie 1951–1955. (Cancer morbidity and mortality in Poland in 1951–1955). *Nowotwory* 10, 55, 1960.
18. *Biuletyn Statystyczny* (Statistical Bulletin). Seria L., Nr 23, GUS, Warszawa, 1964.
19. Bojanowicz K., Gwóźdź B., Sosiński R., Hankiewicz J., Gwóźdź E.: Epidemiologia raka przewodu pokarmowego a uprzemysłowienie i zapylenie powietrza atmosferycznego. (Epidemiology of alimentary tract cancer, and industrialization and air pollution). *Zdr. Publ.* 78, 995, 1967.
20. Boyd J., Langman M., Doll R.: The epidemiology of gastrointestinal cancer with special reference to causation. *GUT*, 5, 3, 1964.

21. Bremmer C. G., Ackerman L. V.: Polyps and carcinoma of the large bowel in the South African Bantu. *Cancer* 26, 991, 1970.

22. Buckwalter J.: Relationship between ABO blood groups and carcinoma of the alimentary tract. In: *Carcinoma of the Alimentary Tract*, W. J. Burdette, ed., University of Utah Press, Salt Lake City, 1965, p 145.

23. Bulbrook R. D.: *Hormones and human breast cancer*. Annual Report and Account, Imperial Cancer Research Fund., London, 1968.

24. Burdette W. J.: Relationship between adenomatous polyps and adenocarcinoma of the colon. In: *Carcinoma of the Alimentary Tract*. W. J. Burdette, ed., University of Utah Press, Salt Lake City, 1965, p. 121.

25. Carrol K. K., Gammal E. B., Plunkett E. R.: Dietary fat and mammary cancer. *Canad. Med. Ass. J.* 98, 590, 1968.

26. Carrol R. E., Haddon W. Jr., Handy V. H., Wieben E. E., Sr.: Thyroid cancer: Cohort analysis of increasing incidence in New York State, 1941–1962. *J. Nat. Cancer Inst.* 33, 277, 1964.

27. Chaklin A. V.: Geographical differences in distribution of malignant tumors. *Bull. Wld. Hlth. Org.*, 27, 337, 1962.

28. Ciechanowski S.: *Nowotwory złośliwe w materiale sekcyjnym Zakładu Anatomii Patologicznej UJ*. (Cancer in the autopsy material of the Department of Pathological Anatomy of the Jagellonian University). Rozprawy Wydz. Lek. Tom 9, PAU, Kraków, 1948.

29. Clemmesen J.: *Statistical Studies in the Aetiology of Malignant Neoplasms*. I. Review and Results. II. Basic Tables, Denmark 1943–1957. Munksgaard, Copenhagen, 1964.

30. Cook P. J., Doll R., Fellingham S. A.: A mathematical model for the age distribution of cancer in man. *Int. J. Cancer* 4, 93, 1969.

31. Correa P., Cuello C., Duque E.: Carcinoma and intestinal metaplasia of the stomach in Colombian migrants. *J. Nat. Cancer Inst.* 44, 297, 1970.

32. Correa P.: Geographic pathology of cancer in Colombia. *Int. Path.* 1, 16, 1970.

33. Correa P.: personal information, 1971.

34. Cutler S. J.: Trends in cancers of the digestive tract. *Surgery* 65, 740, 1969.

35. Cutler S. J., Connelly R. R.: Mammary cancer trends. *Cancer* 23, 767, 1969.

36. Dennis C.: Cancer of the colon and ulcerative colitis. In: *Carcinoma of the Alimentary Tract*. W. J. Burdette, ed., University of Utah Press, Salt Lake City, 1965, p. 157.

37. Doll R.: Worldwide distribution of gastrointestinal cancer. *Nat. Cancer Inst. Monogr.* 25, 174, 1967.

38. Doll R.: The age distribution of cancer in man. In: *Cancer and Aging*. Thule International Symposia, Stockholm, 1968.

39. Doll R.: The geographical distribution of cancer. *Brit. J. Cancer* 23, 1, 1969.

40. Doll R.: Practical steps towards the prevention of bronchial carcinoma. *Scot. Med. J.*, 15, 433, 1970.

41. Doll R., Muir C. S., Waterhouse J. A. H., editors: *Cancer Incidence in Five Continents*. Vol. II, Geneva, UICC, 1970.

42. Dorn H.: Underlying and contributory causes of death. *Nat. Cancer Inst. Monogr.* 19, 421, 1966.

43. Dungal N.: The special problem of stomach cancer in Iceland, with particular reference to dietary factors. *JAMA* 178, 1961.

44. Dunn J. E. Jr., Martin P. L.: Morphogenesis of cervical cancer. Findings from San Diego County cytology registry, *Cancer* 20, 1899, 1967.

45. Eysenck H. J.: *Smoking, Health and Personality*. Weidenfeld and Nicholson, London, 1965.

46. Feinleib M.: Breast cancer and artificial menopause: A cohort study. *J. Nat. Cancer Inst.* 41, 315, 1968.

47. Feinleib M., Garrison R. J.: Interpretation of the vital statistics of breast cancer. *Cancer* 24, 1109, 1969.

48. Flamant R., Lasserre O., Lazar P., Leguerinais J., Denoix P., Schwartz D.: Differences in sex ratio according to cancer site and possible relationship with use of tobacco and alcohol. Review of 65,000 cases. *J. Nat. Cancer Inst.* 32, 1309, 1964.

49. Fraumeni J. F., Jr., Lloyd J. W., Smith E. M., Wagoner J. K.: Cancer mortality among nuns: Role of marital status in etiology of neoplastic disease in women. *J. Nat. Cancer Inst.* 42, 455, 1969.

50. Fraumeni J. F., Jr., Miller R. W.: Leukemia mortality: Downturn rates in the U.S.A., *Science*, 155, 1126, 1967.

51. Freudenberg K.: Hat der Krebs zugenommen? (Has cancer increased?). *Strahlentherapie, Sonderband* 41, 311, 1959.

52. Gadomska H., Karewicz Z.: Zapadalność na raka szyjki macicy na terenie m.st. Warszawy w latach 1963–1967. (Uterine cervix cancer incidence in Warszawa City in 1963–1967). *Gin. Pol.* 41, 1269, 1970.

53. Gordon T., Crittenden M., Haenszel W.: Cancer mortality trends in the United States, 1930–1955. *Nat. Cancer Inst. Monogr.* 6, 133, 1961.

54. Graham S., Levin M., Lilienfeld A. M.: The socioeconomic distribution of cancer of various sites in Buffalo, N.Y., 1948–1952. *Cancer* 13, 180, 1960.

55. Graham S., Levin M. L., Lilienfeld A. M., Sheehe P.: Ethnic derivation as related to cancer at various sites. *Cancer* 16, 13, 1963.

56. Graham S., Lilienfeld A. M., Tidings J. W.: Dietary and purgation factors in the epidemiology of gastric cancer *Cancer* 20, 2224, 1967.

57. Griffith W. G.: The sex ratio in gastric cancer and hypothetical considerations relative to aetiology. *Brit. J. Cancer* 22, 163, 1968.

58. Gsell O.: Trend der Carcinomsterblichkeit der letzten 50–60 Jahre, dargestellt am Beispiel der Schweiz. (Trend of cancer mortality in the last 50–60 years, presented on the example of Switzerland). *Z. Krebsforsch.* 72, 197, 1969.

59. Haenszel W.: Variation in incidence of and mortality from stomach cancer, with particular reference to the United States. *J. Nat. Cancer Inst.* 21, 213, 1958.

60. Haenszel W.: Cancer mortality among the foreign-born in the United States. *J. Nat. Cancer Inst.* 26, 37, 1961.

61. Haenszel W.: Report of the working group on studies of cancer and related diseases in migrant populations. *Int. J. Cancer* 4, 364, 1970.

62. Haenszel W.: personal information.

63. Haenszel W., Correa P.: Cancer of the colon and rectum and adenomatous polyps. *Cancer* 28, 14, 1971.

64. Haenszel W., Dawson E. A.: A note on mortality from cancer of the colon and rectum in the United States. *Cancer* 18, 265, 1965.

65. Haenszel W., Kurihara M.: Studies of Japanese migrants. I. Mortality from cancer and other diseases among Japanese in the United States. *J. Nat. Cancer Inst.* 40, 43, 1968.

66. Haenszel W., Kurihara M., Segi M., Lee R. K. C.: Stomach cancer among Japanese in Hawaii. *J. Nat. Cancer Inst.* 49, 969, 1972.

67. Haenszel W., Loveland D. B., Sirken M. G.: Lung cancer mortality as related to residence and smoking histories. I. White males. *J. Nat. Cancer Inst.* 28, 947, 1962.

68. Haenszel W., Taeuber K. E.: Lung cancer mortality as related to residence and smoking histories. II. White females *J. Nat. Cancer Inst.* 32, 803, 1964.

69. Hakama M., Saxen E. A.: Cereal consumption and gastric cancer. *Int. J. Cancer* 2, 265, 1967.

70. Harvald B., Hauge M.: Heredity of cancer elucidated by a study of unselected twins. *JAMA* 186, 749, 1963.

71. Heasman M. A., Lipworth L.: *Accuracy of certification of cause of death.* General Register Office, London, 1966.

72. Hems G.: Epidemiological characteristics of breast cancer in middle and late age. *Brit. J. Cancer* 24, 226, 1970.

73. Higginson J.: Etiological factors in gastrointestinal cancer in man. *J. Nat. Cancer Inst.* 37, 527, 1966.

74. Higginson J.: Environment and cancer. *Practitioner* 198, 621, 1967.

75. Higginson J.: The theoretical possibilities of cancer prevention in man. *Proc. Roy. Soc. Med.* 61, 723, 1968.

76. Hill B. A.: *Statystyka dla lekarzy.* (Medical Statistics). PWN, Warszawa, 1961.

77. Hiryama T., Wynder E. L.: A study of the epidemiology of cancer of the breast. II. The influence of hysterectomy. *Cancer* 15, 28, 1962.

78. Holzer J. Z.: *Demografia* (Demography). PWE, Warszawa, 1970.

79. International symposium on end results of cancer therapy. *Nat. Cancer Inst. Monogr.* 15, 1964.

80. Janus Z. L., Bailar III J. C., Eisenberg H.: Blood group and uterine cancer. *Amer. J. Epidemiol.* 86, 569, 1967.

81. Johnson L. D., Nickerson R. J., Easterday C. I., Stuart R. S., Hertig A. T.: Epidemiologic evidence for the spectrum of change from dysplasia through carcinoma in situ to invasive cancer. *Cancer* 22, 901, 1968.

82. Jussawalla D. J., Haenszel W., Deshpande V. A., Natekar M. V.: Cancer incidence in Greater Bombay: Assessment of the cancer risk by age. *Brit. J. Cancer* 22, 623, 1968.

83. Just J., Maziarka S., Wyszyńska H.: Badania składu i właściwości rakotwórczych substancji zawartych w pyle zawieszonym w powietrzu atmosferycznym. (Investigations on the composition and carcinogenic properties of substances contained in the dust suspended in the atmosphere air). *Roczn. PZH* 18, 637, 1967.

84. King H., Diamond E., Lilienfeld A. M.: Some epidemiological aspects of cancer of the prostate. *J. chron. Dis.* 16, 117, 1963.

85. Kinosita R., Ishiko T., Sugiyama S., Seto T., Igarasi S., Goetz J. E.: Mycotoxins in fermented food. *Cancer Res.* 28, 2296, 1968.

86. Klebba A. J.: Mortality from selected causes by marital status. United States. Part A. National Center for Health Statistics, Series 20, No. 8a, 1970.

87. Kmet J., Damjanowski L., Stucin M., Bonta S., Čakmakov A.: Circumcision and carcinoma colli uteri in Macedonia, Yugoslavia. Results from a field study. *Brit. J. Cancer* 17, 391, 1963.

88. Kołodziejska H.: Zachorowalność na nowotwory złośliwe w regionie krakowskim w zależności od miejsca zamieszkania. (Cancer incidence by residence in the Kraków Region). *Nowotwory* 20, 305, 1970.

89. Kołodziejska H.: Cancer incidence in Poland, Cracow City and District 1965–66. In: Doll R., Muir C. S., Waterhouse J. A. H., editors: *Cancer Incidence in Five Continents.* Volume II. Geneva, UICC, 1970.

90. Kołodziejska H., Staszewski J., Warda B.: Cancer incidence in Poland, four rural areas, 1965–66. In: Doll R., Muir C. S., Waterhouse J. A. H., editors: *Cancer Incidence in Five Continents.* Volume II. Geneva, UICC, 1970.

91. Kołodziejska H., Strzeszyński J., Nosek H.: Zachorowalność na raka sutka w regionie krakowskim. (Breast cancer incidence in the Kraków Region), *Nowotwory* 15, 317, 1965.

92. Kostrzewski J., Brzeziński Z. J.: Cele, metody i organizacja badań epidemiologicznych w chorobach społecznych. (Aims, methods and organization of epidemiologic studies in social diseases). *Pol. Tyg. Lek.* 25, 421, 1970.

93. Koszarowski T.: O raku płuca — po 25 latach. (On lung cancer — after 25 years). *Pol. Tyg. Lek.* 26, 1805.

94. Koszarowski T.: Cancer incidence in Poland 1965–66. The Polish registries. In: Doll R., Muir C. S., Waterhouse J. A. H., editors: *Cancer Incidence in Five Continents.* Volume II, Geneva, UICC, 1970.

95. Koszarowski T.: Cancer incidence in Poland, Warsaw City, 1965–66. In: Doll R., Muir C. S., Waterhouse J. A. H., editors: *Cancer Incidence in Five Continents.* Volume II. Geneva, UICC, 1970.

96. Koszarowski T.: personal information, 1971.

97. Koszarowski T., Gadomska H.: Wstępne dane o epidemiologii nowotworów złośliwych w Polsce w latach 1952–1962. (Preliminary data on cancer epidemiology in Poland in 1952–1962). *Pol. Tyg. Lek.* 20, 1347, 1965.

98. Koszarowski T., Gadomska H., Warda B., Drożdżewska Z.: *Badania zapadalności i umieralność na nowotwory złośliwe w Polsce i w terenach wybranych 1962–1965.* (Studies of cancer incidence and mortality in Poland and in the selected areas in 1962–1965). PZWL, Warszawa, 1968.

99. Koszarowski T., Kołodziejska H., Gadomska H., Staszewski J., Wieczorkiewicz A., Karewicz Z., Warda B.: Epidemiologia chorób nowotworowych w Polsce w latach 1965–1967. (Epidemiology of cancer in Poland in 1965–1967). *Pol. Tyg. Lek.* 25, 440, 1970.

100. Koszarowski T., Kołodziejska H., Gadomska H., Staszewski J., Wieczorkiewicz A., Karewicz Z., Warda B.: *Epidemiology of neoplasm diseases in Poland, especially in selected areas in the years 1965–1967.* Warszawa, 1970.

101. Kotin P.: Role of migrant populations in studies of environmental effects. *J. Chron. Dis.* 23, 293, 1970.

102. Krasuska W.: Zgony z powodu nowotworów w Warszawie. (Cancer deaths in Warszawa). *Zdr. Publ.* 4, 251, 1966.

103. Kraybill H. F.: Food contaminants and gastrointestinal or liver neoplasia. Survey of experimental observations. *Environm. Res.* 2, 231, 1969.

104. Kreyberg L.: *Histological Lung Cancer Types. A Morphological and Biological Correlation.* Norwegian Universities Press, Oslo, 1962.

105. Kulig A., Jaszcz W., Perski R.: Malignant tumors in the autopsy material of the Department of Pathological Anatomy of the Medical Academy in Cracow in the years 1939–1958. Part I. *Acta Med. Polona* 5, 119, 1964.

106. Laqueur G. L., Spatz M.: Toxicology of Cycasin. *Cancer Res.* 28, 2262, 1968.

107. Laurén P.: The two histological main types of gastric carcinoma: diffuse and so-called intestinal-type carcinoma. An attempt at a histo-clinical classification. *Acta Path. et Microbiol. Scandinav.* 64, 31, 1965.

108. Leńczyk M., Oszacki J., Nosek H.: Badania porównawcze nad rakiem żołądka. (Comparative studies on stomach cancer). *Nowotwory* 16, 265, 1966.

109. Lilienfeld A. M., Pedersen E., Dowd J. E.: *Cancer Epidemiology: Methods of Study.* The John Hopkins Press, Baltimore, 1967.

110. Logan W. P. D.: Marriage and childbearing in relation to cancer of the breast and uterus. *Lancet* 2 (6797), 1199, 1953.

111. Luciak M.: *Zagadnienie raka ukrytego gruczołu krokowego.* (Problem of the occult prostatic cancer). Śląska Akademia Medyczna, 1969.

112. Lundin F. E., Lloyd J. W., Smith E. M., Archer V. E., Holaday D. A.: Mortality of uranium miners in relation to radiation exposure, hard-rock mining and cigarette smoking — 1950 through September 1967. *Health Phys.* 16, 571, 1969.

113. MacMahon B.: Epidemiology of Hodgkin's disease. *Cancer Res.* 26-I, 1180, 1966.

114. MacMahon B., Austin J. H.: Association of carcinomas of the breast and corpus uteri. *Cancer* 23, 275, 1969.

115. MacMahon B., Lin T. M., Lowe C. R., Mirra A. P., Ravnihar B., Salber E. J., Trichopoulos D., Valaoras V. G., Yuasa S.: Lactation and cancer of the breast. A summary of an international study. *Bull. Wld Health Org.* 42, 185, 1970.

116. MacMahon B., Pugh T. F., Ipsen J.: *Epidemiologic Methods.* Little, Brown and Co., Boston, 1960.

117. Mantel N., Haenszel W.: Statistical aspects of the analysis of data from retrospective studies of disease. *J. Nat. Cancer Inst.* 22, 719, 1959.

118. McKenzie A., Case R. A. M., Pearson J. T.: *Cancer statistics for England and Wales, 1901–1955.* General Register Office, London, 1957.

119. Merkov A. M., Tserkownii G. F., Kaufman B. D.: *Morbidity and Mortality from Malignant Neoplasms in the U.S.S.R.* Pitman Medical Publishing Co., London, 1963.

120. *Międzynarodowa klasyfikacja chorób, urazów i przyczyn zgonów,* t. I. (International classification of diseases, injuries and causes of deaths, vol. 1). PZWL, Warszawa, 1960.

121. Mirvish S. S.: Kinetics of nitrosamide formation from alkylureas, N-alkylurethans, and alkylguanidines: possible implications for the etiology of human gastric cancer. *J. Nat. Cancer Inst.* 46, 1183, 1971.

122. Mogilnicki W., Tarłowska L.: Rozkład grup krwi układu ABO u chorych na raka macicy. (Distribution of ABO blood groups in uterus cancer patients). *Nowotwory* 14, 335, 1964.

123. Moriyama I. M., Baum W. S., Haenszel W. M., Mattison B. F.: Inquiry into diagnostic evidence supporting medical certifications of death. *AJPH* 48, 1376, 1958.

124. *Mortality from Malignant Neoplasms,* 1955–1965. Part I, II, WHO, Geneva, 1970.

125. Muñoz N., Asvall J.: Time trends of intestinal and diffuse types of gastric cancer in Norway. *Int. J. Cancer* 8, 144, 1971.

126. Muñoz N., Connelly R.: Time trends of intestinal and diffuse types of gastric cancer in the United States. *Int. J. Cancer* 8, 158, 1971.

127. Muñoz N., Correa P., Cuello C., Duque E.: Histologic types of gastric carcinoma in high- and low-risk areas. *Int. J. Cancer* 3, 809, 1968.

128. Naib Z. M., Nahmias A. J., Josey W. E., Kramer J. H.: Genital herpetic infection. *Cancer* 23, 940, 1969.

129. *Narodowy Spis Powszechny 8.12.1970.* Wyniki ostateczne. Ludność. Zeszyt Nr 23. GUS, Warszawa 1972.

130. National Center for Health Statistics, Washington, D. C.: unpublished data, 1970.

131. Pedersen E.: The presymptomatic diagnosis of cancer: cervix uteri and breast. *Proc. Roy. Soc. Med.* 1189, 1966.

132. Pedersen E., Magnus K.: Gastro-intestinal cancer in Norway. *Acta Un. Int. Cancer* 17, 373, 1961.

133. Pott P.: *Chirurgical observations.* London. 1775.

134. Rawls W. E., Tompkins W. A. F., Melnick J. L.: The association of herpesvirus type 2 and carcinoma of the uterine cervix. *Amer. J. Epidemiol.* 89, 547, 1969.

135. Rees K. R.: Aflatoxin. *GUT*, 7, 205, 1966.

136. Reid B. L.: Cancer of the cervix uteri: review of causal factors with an hypothesis as to its origin. *Med. J. Australia* 1, 375, 1965.

137. Reid B. L.: The possible association of the nucleic acid of sperm in the induction of cervical neoplasia. *Cancer Cytol.* 8, 24, 1968.
138. *Rocznik Statystyczny 1961* (Statistical Yearbook 1961) GUS, Warszawa, 1961.
139. *Rocznik Statystyczny 1970* (Statistical Yearbook 1970) GUS, Warszawa, 1970.
140. *Rocznik Statystyczny 1972* (Statistical Yearbook 1972) GUS, Warszawa, 1972.
141. *Rocznik Statystyczny Ochrony Zdrowia 1945–1967.* (Health Services Statistical Yearbook, 1945–1967). GUS, Warszawa, 1969.
142. Rotkin I. D.: Adolescent coitus and cervical cancer: Associations of related events with increased risk. *Cancer Res.* 27, 603, 1967.
143. Rotkin I. D.: Studies on the inheritance of cancer of the human uterine cervix. *Cancer* 14, 179, 1961.
144. Rotkin I. D.: Further studies in cervical cancer inheritance. *Cancer* 19, 1251, 1966.
145. Rotkin I. D.: Are ABO and Rh blood groups associated with cancer of the uterine cervix? *Cancer* 18, 391, 1965.
146. Rowe N. H., Grammer F. C., Watson F. R., Nickerson N. H.: A study of environmental influence upon salivary gland neoplasia in rats. *Cancer* 26, 436, 1970.
147. Sablińska B., Cieślak M.: Liczne porody jako czynnik usposabiający do zachorowania na raka szyjki macicy u kobiet młodych. (Multiparity as a factor predisposing to uterine cervical cancer in young women). *Nowotwory* 17, 263, 1967.
148. Safiotti U.: Role of vitamin A in carcinogenesis. *Amer. J. Clin. Nutr.* 22, 1088, 1969.
149. Salber E. J., Trichopoulos D., MacMahon B.: Lactation and reproductive histories of breast cancer patients in Boston, 1965–66, *J. Nat. Cancer Inst.* 43, 1013, 1969.
150. Sato T.: Chronic diseases suspected to arise through the enhanced activity of growth hormone by excessive intake of animal protein. III. Corporal cancer and its relation to cervical cancer. *Bull. Inst. Publ. Health* 12, 213, 1963.
151. Sato T.: Chronic diseases suspected to arise through the enhanced activity of growth hormone by excessive intake of animal protein. IV. The cancer and the hypertrophy of the prostate. *Bull. Inst. Publ. Health* 12, 222, 1963.
152. Sato T., Ezaki H.: Studies of the causation of gastric cancer, 4. The distribution of gastric cancer and the intake level of salted foods in Kyushu. *Bull. Inst. Publ. Health* 13, 218, 1964.
153. Sato T., Tsaumuji Y.: Chronic diseases suspected to arise through the enhanced activity of growth hormone by excessive intake of animal protein. II. Breast cancer. *Bull. Inst. Publ. Health* 12, 207, 1963.
154. Schoenberg B. S., Greenberg R. A., Eisenberg H.: Occurrence of certain multiple primary cancers in females. *J. Nat. Cancer Inst.* 43, 15, 1969.
155. Schneider R.: Comparison of age, sex, and incidence rates in human and canine breast cancer. *Cancer* 26, 419, 1970.
156. Schottenfeld D., Berg J.: Incidence of multiple primary cancers. IV. Cancers of the female breast and genital organs. *J. Nat. Cancer Inst.* 46, 161, 1971.
157. Schottenfeld D., Houde R. W.: The changing pattern of cancer morbidity and mortality and its implications. *Medical Clinics of North America* 50, 613, 1966.
158. Schottenfeld D., Lilienfeld A. M., Diamond H.: Some observations on the epidemiology of breast cancer among males. *Amer. J. Public Health* 53, 890, 1963.
159. Segi M., Fukushima I., Fujisaku S., Kurihara M., Saito S., Asano K., Kamoi M.: *Epidemiological study on cancer in Japan.* Gann 48 (Suppl.), 1957.
160. Segi M., Kurihara M.: *Cancer Mortality for Selected Sites in 24 Countries. No. 4 (1962–1963).* Department of Public Health, Tohoku University School of Medicine, Sendai, 1966.

161. Segi M., Kurihara M., Matsuyama T.: *Cancer Mortality for Selected Sites in 24 Countries. No. 5 (1964–1965)*. Department of Public Health, Tohoku University School of Medicine, Sendai, 1970.

162. Selikoff I. J., Hammond E. C., Churg J.: Asbestos exposure, smoking, and neoplasia. *JAMA* 204, 106, 1968.

163. Sigurjonsson J.: Trends in mortality from cancer, with special reference to gastric cancer in Iceland. *J. Nat. Cancer Inst.* 36, 899, 1966.

164. Słomska J.: *Epidemiologia raka szyjki macicy: na podstawie badań własnych*. Praca doktorska. (Epidemiology of uterine cervical cancer: results of a case-control study. Doctoral Thesis). Instytut Onkologii, Gliwice, 1972.

165. *Smoking and Health. Report of the Advisory Committee to the Surgeon General of the Public Health Service*. Public Health Service Publication No. 1103, Washington, 1964.

166. Spiegelman M.: *Introduction to Demography*. Harvard University Press, Cambridge, Mass., 1969.

167. Staszewski J.: Znaczenie palenia tytoniu w powstawaniu raka oskrzeli. (Smoking habits and bronchial carcinoma). *Pol. Tyg. Lek.* 14, 1904, 1959.

168. Staszewski J.: Smoking and cancer in Poland. *Brit. J. Cancer* 14, 419, 1960.

169. Staszewski J.: Umieralność z powodu nowotworów złośliwych w Polsce w 1959 r. (Cancer mortality in Poland in 1959). *Nowotwory* 14, 63, 1964.

170. Staszewski J.: Regionalne różnice rejestracji umieralności na nowotwory w Polsce w 1961 r. (Regional differences of cancer mortality in Poland in 1961). *Nowotwory* 17, 297, 1967.

171. Staszewski J.: Wartość statystyk zgonów w badaniach nad epidemiologią nowotworów złośliwych. (The value of mortality statistics in research on cancer epidemiology). *Nowotwory* 17, 371, 1967.

172. Staszewski J.: Umieralność na raka płuc w Polsce a palenie tytoniu i zanieczyszczenia atmosfery (Lung cancer mortality, smoking and air pollution in Poland). *Przegl. Epid.* 22, 131, 1968.

173. Staszewski J.: Próba oceny wpływu niektórych czynników na występowanie raka sutka wśród kobiet w Polsce. (An evaluation of the correlation of some factors with the distribution of female breast cancer in Poland). *Nowotwory* 18, 295, 1968.

174. Staszewski J.: Smoking and cancer of the alimentary tract in Poland. *Brit. J. Cancer* 23, 247, 1969.

175. Staszewski J.: Apropos of summarizing indices for comparison of cancer incidence data. *Neoplasma* 16, 321, 1969.

176. Staszewski J.: Wzrost umieralności na raka sutka wśród kobiet w Polsce. (Increase in breast cancer mortality in Poland). *Nowotwory* 20, 311, 1970.

177. Staszewski J.: Rola statystyki zgonów w badaniach epidemiologii nowotworów w Polsce. (Role of mortality statistics in research on cancer epidemiology in Poland). *Pol. Tyg. Lek.* 26, 225, 1971.

178. Staszewski J.: Odżywianie a rak żołądka (Dietary habits and stomach cancer). *Nowotwory* 21, 119, 1971.

179. Staszewski J.: Age at menarche and breast cancer. *J. Nat. Cancer Inst.* 47, 935, 1971.

180. Staszewski J., Haenszel W.: Cancer mortality among the Polish-born in the United States. *J. Nat. Cancer Inst.* 35, 291, 1965.

181. Staszewski J., McCall M., Stenhouse N. S.: Cancer mortality in 1962–1966 among Polish migrants to Australia. *Brit. J. Cancer* 25, 599, 1971.

182. Staszewski J., Muir C. S., Słomska J., Jain K.: Sources of demographic data on migrant groups for epidemiological studies of chronic diseases. *J. Chron. Dis.* 23, 351, 1970.

183. Staszewski J., Niepołomska W.: Opracowanie rozpoznań histopatologicznych w materiale rejestru nowotworów. (Evaluation of histopathologic data in cancer registry). *Pol. Tyg. Lek.* 24, 1936, 1969.

184. Staszewski J., Słomska J.: Regionalne różnice umieralności z powodu raka macicy a płodność i wiek zamążpójścia. (Regional differences in uterine cancer mortality in Poland related to fertility and to age at marriage). *Nowotwory* 18, 77, 1968.

185. Staszewski J., Słomska J.: Płodność kobiet a najczęstsze umiejscowienie nowotworów. (Fertility and the most frequent female cancers). *Gin. Pol.* 42, 359, 1971.

186. *Statystyka Ludności. Małżeństwa, urodzenia, zgony, 1960.* (Vital Statistics: Marriages, births, deaths). GUS, Warszawa 1964.

187. Stemmermann G. N.: Patterns of disease among Japanese living in Hawaii. *Arch. Environ. Health* 20, 266, 1970.

188. Stemmermann G. N.: personal communication, 1970.

189. Stern R. (1844) — cited after [29].

190. Stocks P.: Cancer of the uterine cervix and social conditions. *Brit. J. Cancer* 9, 487, 1955.

191. Stocks P.: Social status in relation to carcinoma of the breast. *Schweiz. Z. Path. Bakt.* 18, 706, 1955.

192. Stocks P., Davies R. I.: Zinc and copper content of soils associated with the incidence of cancer of the stomach and cther organs. *Brit. J. Cancer* 18, 14, 1964.

193. Tanner J. M.: *Rozwój w okresie pokwitania.* (Growth at adolescence). PZWL, Warszawa, 1963.

194. Terris M., Hall C. E.: Decline in mortality from gastric cancer in native-born and foreign-born residents of New York City. *J. Nat. Cancer Inst.* 31, 155, 1963.

195. *The Cancer Registry of Norway: Trends in Cancer Incidence in Norway 1955–1967.* Universitetsforlaget, 1972.

196. *The Health Consequences of Smoking. A Public Health Service Review:* 1967, and 1968 Supplement. Public Health Service Publication No. 1966, Washington 1967, and 1968.

197. *The Registrar General's Decennial Supplement, England and Wales,* 1951, *Occupational Mortality.* Part II. Vol. 1: Commentary, vol. 2: Tables. General Register Office, London, 1958.

198. Toman R., Gregor O., Drnkov'a V., Pasterová J.: Geographical differences in the incidence of gastric carcinoma in Czechoslovakia. *Vnitřni lèkařstvi* 12, 994, 1966.

199. *Umieralność w latach 1958–1969.* (Mortality in 1958–1969). GUS, Warszawa, 1971.

200. *Umieralność według przyczyn w latach 1951–1970.* (Mortality by cause in 1951–1970). GUS, Warszawa, 1972.

201. Urban A.: Morfologia wrzodu żołądka i współistniejących z nim zmian strukturalnych śluzówki. (Morphology of stomach ulcer and of the co-existing structural lesions of mucosa). *Folia Medica Cracoviensis* 2, 223, 1960.

202. Valaoras V. G., MacMahon B., Trichopoulos D., Polychronopoulou A.: Lactation and reproductive histories of breast cancer patients in Greater Athens 1965–1967. *Int. J. Cancer* 4, 350, 1969.

203. Waard de F.: Adrenal oestrogen and the geographical distribution of breast cancer. *Achtiende Jaarboek van Kankeronderzoek en Nederland,* 191, 1968.

204. Waard de F.: The epidemiology of breast cancer; review and prospects. *Int. J. Cancer* 4, 577, 1969.

205. Wahi P. N., Mali S., Luthra U. K.: Factors influencing cancer of the uterine cervix in North India. *Cancer* 23, 1221, 1969.

206. Wieczorkiewicz A., Staszewski J.: Cancer incidence in Poland in Katowice District. In: Doll R., Muir C. S., Waterhouse J. A. H., editors: *Cancer incidence in Five Continents*. Volume II. Geneva, UICC, 1970.

207. Winter K.: Die Akzeleration als Ausdruck der gesellschaftlich bedingten Wandlung der Biologie des Menschen. (Acceleration as an expression of the socially related changes in human biology). *Zschr. ärztl. Fortbild*. 58, 1101, 1964.

208. Wynder E. L.: Identification of women at high risk for breast cancer. *Cancer* 24, 1235, 1969.

209. Wynder E. L.: personal information.

210. Wynder E. L., Bross I. J.: A study of etiological factors in cancer of the esophagus. *Cancer* 14, 389, 1961.

211. Wynder E. L., Bross I. J., Hirayama T.: A study of the epidemiology of cancer of the breast. *Cancer* 13, 559, 1960.

212. Wynder E. L., Escher G. C., Mantel N.: An epidemiological investigation of cancer of the endometrium. *Cancer* 19, 489, 1966.

213. Wynder E. L., Graham S., Eisenberg H.: Conference on the etiopathology of cancer of the gastro-intestinal tract. *Cancer* 19, 1561, 1966.

214. Wynder E. L., Hyams L., Shigematsu T.: Correlation of international cancer death rates: An epidemiological exercise. *Cancer* 20, 113, 1967.

215. Wynder E. L., Kajitani T., Ishikawa S., Dodo H., Takano A.: Environmental factors of cancer of the colon and rectum. II. Japanese epidemiological data. *Cancer* 23, 1210, 1969.

216. Wynder E. L., Kajitani T., Kuno J., Lucas J. C., De Palo A., Farrow J.: A comparison of survival rates between American and Japanese patients with breast cancer. *Surg. Gynecol. Obstet*. 117, 196, 1963.

217. Wynder E. L., Kmet J., Dungal N., Segi M.: An epidemiological investigation of gastric cancer. *Cancer* 16, 1461, 1963.

218. Wynder E. L., Shigematsu T.: Environmental factors of cancer of the colon and rectum. *Cancer* 20, 1520, 1967.

219. *Wyniki badania struktury ludności według płci i wieku. Stan w dniu 31.12.1967 r*. (Results of the study of the structure of population by sex and age as of 31 December 1967). GUS, Warszawa, 1969.

220. Yuasa S., MacMahon B.: Lactation and reproductive histories of breast cancer patients in Tokyo, Japan. *Bull. WHO* 42, 195, 1970.

221. Zacharias L., Wurtman R. J.: Age at menarche. *New Eng. J. Med*. 280, 868, 1969.

Index

* they *are*: Breast, Intestinal tract, Lung, Prostate, Stomach, and Uterus cancers. *See also* Other cancers mentioned

** *such as* Aflatoxins, Air pollution, Alcohol, Aniline dyes, Arsen, Asbestos, Biliary salts, Bittner's milk factor, Chromium, Herpesvirus, Ionizing radiation, Nickel, Nitrogen mustard, Nitrosamines, Tobacco, Uranium ores, Water pollutants

* (C) — the catchword relates specifically to cervical carcinoma
** (E) — the catchword relates specifically to corporal (endometrial) carcinoma